THE ALL NEW AMERICAN DIET

TODD D. GLASSMAN, D.O.

THE ALL NEW AMERICAN DIET

You should not undertake any diet/exercise regimen recommended in this book
before consulting your personal physician. Neither the author nor the publisher shall
be responsible or liable for any loss or damage allegedly arising as a consequence of
your use or application of any information or suggestions contained in this book.

iUniverse books may be ordered through booksellers or by contacting:

iUniverse LLC
1663 Liberty Drive
Bloomington, IN 47403
www.iuniverse.com
1-800-Authors (1-800-288-4677)

Because of the dynamic nature of the Internet, any web addresses or links contained in
this book may have changed since publication and may no longer be valid. The views
expressed in this work are solely those of the author and do not necessarily reflect the
views of the publisher, and the publisher hereby disclaims any responsibility for them.

Any people depicted in stock imagery provided by Thinkstock are models,
and such images are being used for illustrative purposes only.
Certain stock imagery © Thinkstock.

ISBN: 978-1-4917-0797-5 (sc)
ISBN: 978-1-4917-0801-9 (e)

Printed in the United States of America.

iUniverse rev. date: 12/06/2013

Dedication page

To my Mother and Father for their moral support; to my Wife for loving me; to my Daughter for believing in me; to my family, friends, and patients for their inspiration, motivation, and encouragement to finish the book.

Index

Introduction

You know you are too heavy and have to lose weight! You have known this for years. You have tried diets and exercise, but it has not been easy. You have probably given up and are most likely wondering what makes this book any different than the others you have read. The answer is that in this book, I will give you a plan to follow so you can successfully achieve your goals. If you follow the basic principles detailed in these pages—principles that have been tested and proven effective—losing weight can be achieved.

In 2000, I went to see my primary care provider and was diagnosed with hypertension. My blood pressure was 185/90, and my weight was over 190 pounds. This may not seem like a lot of weight but at 5'9", it put my body mass index (the overweight region on the BMI scale) at 29—one point away from obesity. Needless to say, my primary care provider said that I needed to lose weight. I was under a lot of stress at the time, working as a resident physician at Palmetto General Hospital, and my first thought was, "That is impossible." And then I asked myself, "How do I do that?" I had struggled with my weight my entire life, and now I was being told by my doctor to go on the "Zone Diet." Although I had never heard of this diet, I bought the book, read it, and tried to follow it, all without success. I then decided to try the "Adkins Diet." It worked for a while, until I went back to eating carbohydrates and my abdomen blew up like a balloon. Now, instead of 190, I was pushing 200 pounds. I was very frustrated. The diets were not working, and I didn't know what to do.

Since I had successfully done the "Slim Fast Diet" in the past, I decided to try it again, only this time I did my own version of it by using a product called "Soy Slender." It worked! I substituted my breakfast and lunch with a large glass of Soy Slender and had a sensible meal for dinner. I lost weight on this diet and was finally able to enjoy positive results, until I reached a plateau. At 170 pounds, I was still overweight and struggling to reach my goal. I needed to lose 20 more pounds, but I was stuck at that weight. That was when my wife, on her friend's recommendation, suggested that I try the "Jenny Craig" diet. It had worked for them and also for my uncle who had lost a lot of weight on the diet. So, I tried it, and it worked! I reached my goal weight! The small, pre-packaged meals made it easy and convenient to follow the diet. I received counseling on what to eat, when to eat, and how to eat. The program provided good education on proper nutrition, portion control and "volumetrics". These important concepts on dieting will be discussed in further detail in the book. By using these three concepts, weight loss can be achieved. There were weekly meetings and weigh-ins at the center. The support provided by the staff and the literature I read, helped a lot. Six months later, I reached my goal weight of 150 pounds. I lost close to 50 pounds, and my blood pressure finally normalized with my new weight and with the aid of medication. Why did I share my story with you? To inspire you to "never give up." If you want something bad enough, keep trying. If you are truly motivated, you can accomplish your goals.

In this book, I share key concepts to help you reach your goal. Each page is filled with practical information that will give you the knowledge you need to finally reach your ideal body weight—and all the food is easy to prepare! This book is designed to be simple, so anyone can follow the diet. You will also learn the importance of exercise. If you think you can lose weight without exercise, stop reading this book right now. You need both, diet and exercise, to achieve weight loss. When I started my weight loss program, I joined Jenny Craig and L.A. Fitness. By combining the two, I was able to defeat the obesity monster I had been fighting for years.

This journey is similar to a soldier going into battle. If you fight the enemy head on, you will get slaughtered. However, if you attack your enemy from two or three different directions, you are more likely to win the battle. I am not telling you to join L.A. Fitness or any other gym. I know this can be expensive. But there are many ways to exercise without the expense. For example: walk, hike, jog, ride a bike, swim, dance, or aqua aerobics. You can play with your kids or do sports—like softball, baseball, football, basketball, hockey, boxing, or even golf. You can ice skate, snow or water ski, go snorkeling or bowling. You can use an elliptical machine, rowing machine, or a stationary bike. There are many things you can do to become active. The point is to be active. So get up and get your body moving! Motion is the key to life.

Ten Golden Keys
to Diet Success

The success of any diet program depends on many factors, but here are ten golden keys to remember *and* implement when deciding to start a health program.

1. Goals

The first thing you have to do when starting a health program is to set a goal. Begin by establishing what your ideal weight should be for your age by calculating your BMI (Body Mass Index). This formula is used by doctors to diagnose obesity.[1] (See pages 81 - 83 for more information on obtaining your BMI.) Your ideal weight, according to the BMI chart, should be your goal weight. This can be found in the normal BMI range. Once you have that, write it down in a notebook or a diary. You can also meet with a nutritionist or dietician who can help you to record your goals and progress. Do not skip this step. It is very important to set goals, so you can have a beginning and an end. Establishing your goals will give you focus—something to set your sites on and aim for. It will help you set up a plan and stick to it. As you begin to lose weight and you get close to your goal, it will help to motivate you. Don't rush to meet your goal. Take small steps to accomplish it. For example, if you weigh

200 pounds and your goal is to weigh 150 pounds, your first goal should be to lose 25 pounds. When you reach 175 pounds, you will be half way there, and you will feel a sense of accomplishment. Achieving this first goal and seeing your progress in writing and in the mirror will give you a sense of accomplishment. My personal goal was to weigh 150 pounds. I went from 190 plus pounds to 150 pounds in only a few months. Another goal was to keep the weight off, and I have successfully done this because I follow my own advice: I set goals and take small steps to ensure their successful completion.

2. Priority.

You are a very important person. That is why your diet goals should be a priority in your life. You need to make weight loss a priority—the number one thing to accomplish on your to-do list, each day. We are always rushing to get somewhere, and every day we seem to get busier with family and work, but we must focus on what is important. One thing to remember is that some days might present challenges (emergencies) that will compromise our diet goals for the day. On such days, take care of those "unexpected events," and then, the next day, go back to your diet goals, giving them priority.

3. You deserve it.

By now you should know how important you are. You also know that it is important to place dieting high up on your priority list of things to do. Now there are a few more things you need to know: You deserve to take care of yourself. You deserve to eat healthy. You deserve to eat often, and you should not be ashamed to eat. You may not be used to taking care of yourself. You might be one of those people who does every-thing for everyone else. Maybe you're the soccer mom with three kids or the executive taking care of all the employees. But whoever you are, and regardless of what you do, for once in your life, I want you to take care of you. I know this might sound selfish, but it is not because if you do not take care of yourself, you will not be able to take care of anyone else. If you don't take care of yourself, who will do it for you? I want you to eat healthy food. As a matter of fact, you are entitled to eat well, and it is OK to do it! The best thing about the All New American Diet is that you have to eat, and you have to eat often. I know that sounds odd, but that is how it works. That is how you will lose weight: by eating the right types of foods in small portions. Eating often is the secret to weight loss. It is that simple! You need to keep your metabolism revved up, and you do this by eating five or six times a day (small frequent meals). If you only eat one or two meals a day, your body will go into starvation mode. When you do this, you are basically telling your brain, "I don't know when I will eat again," and your body will start to store fat. You need to take time out of your busy schedule to eat. It only takes a few minutes to eat a snack or a meal. You deserve to eat, and you have to eat. So for once in your life, take care of yourself. If you do this, everyone you love will benefit.

4. Think.

You may have heard of the book "Think and Grow Rich." Well, I want you to think and lose weight. My mother always told me, "consciousness, Todd, consciousness." What does that mean? It means that you need to *think* about what you are going to eat, and plan your meals in advance. You need to prepare your own meals. You need to ask yourself, "Should I have that chocolate cake with ice cream?" And then give yourself the answer, "No! I have a goal to keep. My diet desert is at home." You need to think through the temptation. Try this: stop, close your eyes, and take a couple of deep breaths as you remind yourself of your set goals. If you do this, the temptation will pass, in time. Don't fret. The cake and ice cream are not going anywhere. You will enjoy them again, *after* you reach your goals. The urge to eat it "right now" will pass. After you eat the desert allotted in the diet, you will not eat anything else for the rest of the day. Instead, think about what you will have for breakfast the following morning. Think about when you are going out to dinner, and what you can eat that is diet compatible. Think about the football game you plan to go to. What can you eat that will not destroy your diet? Have the grilled chicken sandwich, instead of the Italian sausage. Have the light beer, instead of the regular beer. You need to think, and focus on your diet. This will help you stay on track for your diet goal.

5. Will Power.

What is will power? Webster defines "will power" as "energetic determination."[2] I define it as "your desire and discipline to overcome an obstacle"; "to impose your will on something or someone." Think of will power as the goal of a football team imposing its will on its opponent. Will power requires that you dig deep within yourself to find and harness the energy you will need to stay focus on your goals. How much will power do you have to accomplish your goal? You have it. Everyone does. You just need to do some soul searching to discover it, and then you have to make the decision to use it. I guarantee that it exists inside of you. So find your will power, and get to work!

6. Balance.

Balance is important for successful weight loss. Try to have some balance and not go to extremes when it comes to eating. You want to keep your blood glucose levels even keel throughout the day. You don't want the peaks and valleys of high and low blood glucose. Try to achieve equilibrium with your body's biochemistry.

7. Gifts.

Reward yourself for doing a good job on your diet. Give yourself a gift; perhaps a pair of running shoes. This will motivate you and help you exercise more. Another good gift you will enjoy and help you stay on track with your goals is an iPod. They are perfect for working out. Fill it with inspiring music. You will be surprised how much music could motivate you. Music has a strong, psychological impact on your mind. You can download the music you like off the internet or iTunes. Another example of a perfect gift would be workout clothes. The point is to reward yourself with other items besides food. Joining a gym is also a very beneficial and motivating gift. If you like the outdoors, buy a bike. When you lose weight and reach your goal, you can buy new clothes. Give yourself whatever works to keep you motivated and moving. Be creative! If you like to mow the lawn, get a new lawn mower. If you don't want to spend a lot of money, go to the movies or buy a good book. Better yet, go to the library and check out a book for free. Do whatever works for you. If you lose two or three pounds in one week, reward yourself with a massage. It will loosen up your muscles and make you feel so good, that you will be ready for the following week. Treat yourself because you deserve it. You worked hard for it!

8. Kindness.

Be kind to yourself and others. Don't beat yourself up if you make a mistake on your diet. Don't shame yourself because you ate a piece of chocolate cake, candy, or milkshake. Instead, realize that you made a mistake, and start your diet again at your next meal or the next day.

9. Educate.

You need to constantly educate yourself on weight loss and maintenance. Read books, watch movies, and listen to CDs that will help you learn new ideas and techniques to help you lose weight. This is the information age, and knowledge is power. If you don't have time to read a book, then listen to audio books. Purchase a good audio diet book, and listen to it while driving, doing chores around the house, or when you are walking or doing any activity you enjoy. This will keep you motivated and inspired. Many people have new and different ideas that can help you with your weight loss goals. You have to keep on learning to stay consistent with your diet. If you don't learn new ideas, you will get bored and be tempted to go back to your old habits. If food preparation and portion control is a problem for you, then join a weight loss club like Jenny Craig, Weight Watchers, or Nutrasystem. These are great learning tools to help you lose weight. If you are confused or simply want more information on proper nutrition, consult a certified nutritionist or dietician. They have a wealth of knowledge. You can also hire a personal trainer or simply talk to one and ask about a nutrition plan. You can buy a diet recipe book, go to the public library and check out books on nutrition and dieting, or even go online and download easy-to-prepare meals and recipes.

10. Motivation.

This is everything we just talked about. By understanding the nine other golden keys and applying them, you will become motivated and remain that way until you reach your ideal goal weight. As you see yourself losing weight, your motivation will increase. Knowing that the diet is working will keep you motivated. Buy a scale, and keep it in your bathroom, but only weigh yourself once a week. Try doing it on the same day, every week (e.g. every Friday or every Monday). Pick a day and be consistent. When your clothes begin to fit better, you will not want to stop. Want more motivation? Try watching movies like "Rocky" (the original) or "Vision Quest." Also, think of some phrases to keep you inspired. For example, "Eye of the tiger," "Slow and steady wins the race," and "No pain no gain." "An apple a day keeps the doctor away," "One day at a time," "Eat to live; don't live to eat," "Go to work, and work hard."

Let's recap: Before starting a diet program, you need to set reasonable *goals* and make your decision to lose weight a *priority*. Remember that you are unique and important. You *deserve* to eat healthy, so *think* about what you are going to eat, and plan your meals in advance. Dig deep for the *will power* you will need to stay on track. You have it! It's in you! Establish a *balance* in your new eating habits, but go all out to reward yourself with *gifts* that will motivate you to keep going. Not eating everything your body craves might make you moody, but remember to be *kind* to yourself and others. Do whatever it takes to *educate* yourself on proper nutrition, dieting, and exercise programs. And last but most importantly, don't give up. Fuel your motivation!

Before getting into the program, let me share some alarming numbers with you. Check out the next chapter.

Alarming Numbers

Many people understand their personal need for good nutrition, exercise, and a lifestyle change, but few are truly aware of the seriousness of the situation when it comes to obesity, especially in the United States. Before going any further, here are the results of some studies done in the United States concerning obesity and health. Understanding the problem is part of the solution.

1. In America, almost one in four people die from heart disease. In 2008, more than 615,000 people in the United States died from heart disease. [1]

2. Heart disease is the number one cause of death in the United States.[1]

3. The most common type of heart disease in the United States is coronary heart disease. In 2008, more than 400,000 people in the United States died from coronary heart disease.[1]

4. In 2010, the annual cost for coronary heart disease was estimated to be almost 109 billion dollars.[1]

5. Approximately 1 out of 3 United States citizens has hypertension. The number of individuals is estimated to be 68 million. High blood pressure increases your chances of getting a cerebral vascular accident or heart

disease. The number 1 cause of death in the United States is heart disease. The third cause of death in the United States is a cerebral vascular accident.[2]

6. The three leading causes of death are as follows: Heart disease, cancer, and stroke.[3]

7. The three most common types of cancer in men are as follows: Prostate, lung, and rectum/colon.[4]

8. The three most common types of cancer in women: Breast, lung, and rectum/colon.[5]

9. Over the past forty years, smoking tobacco has decreased by one third. However, over that same time period, obesity has doubled in the United States.[6]

10. Over one third of the United States adult population is obese. Recent data shows an increase of approximately 35% obesity rate in the United States for adults. Some of the leading causes of deaths are directly related to obesity. These include: Heart disease, cancer, stroke, and diabetes. In 2008, the cost associated with obesity was almost 150 billion dollars.[7]

11. Obesity also affects children and teenagers in the United States. The current rate of obesity in this age group is 17%. This rate has tripled over the past 20 years.[8]

12. In 2010, over 25 million people were known to have Diabetes in the United States. This would be approximately 8% of the population.[9]

13. The leading cause of disability in the United States for ages 15 - 44 is major depressive disorder. Almost 15 million American adults are affected by major depressive disorder. This is almost 7% of the United

States population. Major depressive disorder seems to be more common in women. The average age of onset is 32 years old.[10]

14. Osteoarthritis (OA), also known as degenerative joint disease (DJD), affects more than 25 million American adults. One out of every two American adults will develop some form of OA/DJD.[11]

15. Approximately two million Americans are affected by Rheumatoid Arthritis (RA). This disease is more disabling than osteoarthritis (OA). It usually starts at a younger age, and it affects women more than men.[12]

16. Over 50 million adults in the United States suffer from chronic pain. The projected annual cost for chronic pain is approximately 90 billion dollars.[13]

Now that you have an idea of the importance of good nutrition, let us see what we can do to never join these statistics.

Just Eat
Half—Portion Control

When I was 15 years old, my father and I went to see a St. Louis Cardinals Baseball game. Before getting to the game, we decided to get some dinner at a famous Italian restaurant in downtown St. Louis. When it came time to order, he said to me, "Why don't we share a dish, and we will just eat half." That night we shared a dish of linguini with white clam sauce, and the amount of food that we ate was just the right amount. That night was the first time I heard the phrase "just eat half."

In America today, everything is super-sized. If you don't believe me, just turn on your TV and watch the show "Man versus Food." Meal portions served at restaurants are almost always enough for two people. So the next time you decide to enjoy a restaurant meal, split it with a friend, your spouse, or one of your children. If you are single, eat half of the meal, and take the rest home. You can have the leftovers for lunch or for dinner the next day. Fill up on salad, vegetables, and water, and remember to "just eat half," and you will never go wrong.

When I prepare my lunch, I only eat half of it. Make whatever type of sandwich you like, and cut it in half. Eat half the sandwich for one meal, and save the other half for the next meal or the next day. Make sure to bring a medium to large salad or vegetables to go along with your half sandwich. You should also drink one bottle of water with each meal. This will fill you up and leave you feeling satisfied. And don't worry about feeling hungry too soon because, in three hours, you can have a snack.

You will want to get into the habit of eating only half for all of your meals: breakfast, lunch, and dinner. I love sandwiches, so for breakfast, I make one of my favorites: egg sandwich. However, instead of two eggs, I eat only one egg or two egg whites. Instead of two pieces of toast, I eat only one piece. I also add fruit to my breakfast; half an apple instead of a whole apple or half a banana rather than a whole one. Whatever type of fruit you like, "just eat half." If you like grapes or strawberries, eat only half a cup which is approximately what would fit in the palm of your hand. Add some coffee or green tea, with a small amount of skim milk or almond milk, your favorite sweetener, and you are good to go for the morning. My personal preference is adding a small amount of almond milk with one or two packages of Truvia. Just remember to eliminate high calorie foods such as cream and sugar.

As you can see, it is not about denying yourself the joy of eating but about portion control. Everything should be portioned out. The Jenny Craig diet and Lean Cuisine frozen foods are the perfect example of what proper food portions look like. My freezer was always full of these food items. They helped my wife and I to know how much food to eat and to lose weight.

There are no frozen entrees in the diet I am introducing you to. However, you will need to portion out all of your meals.

The best way to start is to purchase small plastic containers, plastic bags, and aluminum foil. You will be preparing most of your meals, and that is a good thing because you will know exactly what you are eating. For lunch and dinner, you will want to eat 2 - 4 oz of protein—about the size of your palm. (2 oz of protein is half the size of your palm.) The carbohydrate intake should be half a cup of rice, pasta, half of a potato, or one slice of whole grain bread. The rest of your meal should be some type of vegetable. If you are still hungry, eat more vegetables. Ideally, vegetables should be raw, steamed, or grilled. You can also microwave vegetables if you are in a hurry. You should never smother your vegetables in cream, cheese, or butter or sauté them in a lot of oil. However, it is OK to use extra virgin olive oil, sparingly.

Prepare your meal using proper portion control and place it in the plastic containers, plastic bags, or wrap it in aluminum foil. Take a bottle of water. (You can use a 16.9 oz water bottle, and try to drink four of these throughout the day.) Use a small plastic container (you can find this at your local grocery store) to take your salad dressing. It is important not to eliminate the dressing because it adds flavor to your salad, and it makes your meal experience much more enjoyable. (Please refer to the grocery list presented later in the book for more choices and portion control.) I suggest using extra virgin olive oil, rice vinegar, and seasoning, or you can use low-fat yogurt dressing; no more than 1 or 2 oz for whichever one you choose. This is an important point to learn because salad dressing can add a lot of calories to your daily intake—using more than the recommended amounts will slow down or stop your weight loss. When ordering at a restaurant, always ask for your salad dressing to be served on the side, and just eat half!

Eat Less and Age Slower

Are you interested in slowing down the aging process and living longer? The media, especially television and internet, is filled with advertisings and marketing campaigns presenting one product or another that promises to prevent or take away wrinkles, make you stronger, smarter, healthier, and even skinnier, but do they really work? Is there a miracle product in the market that can do any of these things? Is there anything we can do to look younger, without the expense of fancy products and empty promises? What if there was something you could do to slow down the aging process and look younger longer. Would you be willing to try? If yes, than here it is: eat right.

Studies have shown that eating less will slow down the aging process. There is a group of people in Okinawa—islands off the coast of Japan—that seem to age slower and live longer than others. After careful observation, it was noted that these people tend to have low calorie diets, which is certainly a big contributor in the statistics that show lower rates of people on the island suffering of heart disease, cancer, and cerebral vascular accidents than the Japanese people. Okinawa has a large number of individuals who live to be 100 years old and older.[1] More human studies need to be conducted.

Anti-aging is a topic that almost everyone is interested in learning more about. By using portion control and calorie restriction, you will age slower. One animal study showed that by decreasing their calorie intake by 40 percent, the animal could extend his life span by almost half. Not only would the animal live longer but also healthier.[1]

How does eating fewer calories slow down the aging process? When you eat, it takes a lot of energy to digest food and then store it away. Many chemical reactions take place during this process. For example, during these chemical reactions, free radicals, which can cause a lot of damage to the microscopic network of the body, are produced. Therefore, eating less produces fewer chemical reactions, which in turn produces less free radicals.[1]

A low calorie diet will also decrease the amount of triglycerides and cholesterol in the blood stream; thus keeping the blood vessels clean and open and allow for smooth blood flow, making the blood less turbulent. The endothelium (the cells that form the inside lining of the blood vessels) can function better without plaque. If the endothelium works efficiently, it can release the chemicals it needs to and primarily release the chemical nitric oxide. Again, this chemical will help dilate blood vessels and allow the blood to flow smoother. This in turn will lower your blood pressure and make it less likely to develop a myocardial infarction or a cerebral vascular accident; both can be life threatening.[1] The heart can also work more efficiently.

In regard to nitric oxide, this is a very important biochemical. It has many biological functions. Nitric oxide will cause vasodilation (the expansion of blood vessels), lowers blood pressure, lowers lipids in the blood, helps stop blood clots from forming, and it helps with neurotransmission.[2] It is very important to keep the arteries and arterioles smooth and clean so that nitric oxide can be released from the endothelium. And you do this by having a healthy diet and exercising regularly. Your doctor may prescribe a medicine classified as a statin. This medicine will help lower cholesterol and keep the blood vessels clean.

Now you know that eating less will most likely slow down the aging process. So keep that in mind the next time you cook or enjoy a night out.

Hormones

When you eat, your body responds by releasing hormones into your blood stream. If you eat a large amount of carbohydrates (for example, a large bowl of pasta), your pancreas will secrete insulin. The insulin will then take the glucose that is in your blood stream and store it away as fat. Insulin has a counter acting hormone called glucagon. This hormone— secreted by the pancreas—has the opposite effect of insulin. Insulin lowers blood glucose levels, and glucagon (stimulated by eating protein) increases blood glucose levels, as well as break down stored glucose in the liver.[1] These two hormones need to be in balance to achieve optimum energy levels that will help you to feel your best. Insulin and glucagon are not the only hormones in your body. Obviously, you have a lot of different types of hormones in your body. Hormones work on multiple body systems. These include: the central nervous system, the cardiovascular system, the endocrine system, the lymphatic system, the musculoskeletal system, and the reproductive system. There are other hormones that work at the cellular level, and eating the right way will help balance these hormones as well.[1] Not only does the food you eat cause your body to secrete hormones, but they give the body the building blocks to form the hormones. In biochemistry, this is known as being in equilibrium.

How do you get equilibrium? By eating small, frequent meals throughout the day and by practicing portion control. Each meal should be eaten every three to four hours, and they should include all the basics: protein, carbohydrate, fat, and fiber. If this is done, your blood chemistry will reach equilibrium, and you will feel great.

On occasion, my wife and I discuss obesity. She says it is all genetic, but I argue saying that it is mostly caused by bad eating habits. Many diseases have a genetic root. These include: heart disease, diabetes, cancer, obesity, addiction, and depression. By eating a low calorie diet that is macronutrient balanced, you greatly decrease the chances of those genes from being activated. The more you indulge and don't monitor your food intake the more likely the disease gene will be activated.[1]

You want your body to burn fat. This is where you get a high energy surge. You do not want to use the stored glucose in your liver or muscle. Remember, fat has double the amount of calories that carbohydrate or protein has, per molecule. By following my diet plan, you will be able to tap into these high energy sources (the fat molecules).

Exercise and the Scientific Data

We have discussed the need to set goals when beginning a new nutrition program and the importance of making this a priority. We know that we are special and deserve to be healthy, and to do this we must think about what we eat and have the will power to persevere and stay on track. We have read some alarming numbers concerning obesity, heart disease, hypertension, and more. We were introduced to the phrase, "eat half", and the importance of portion control. In addition, we know that eating less may slow down the aging process. Finally, we briefly covered the work of hormones in our bodies and the importance of equilibrium for healthy living. Now we will educate ourselves on the importance of exercise. Let us begin with the following scientific data, before going into the heart of the matter. The information you are about to read is important because it will increase your awareness of impending health dangers if you don't make the decision to eat healthy and exercise.

"**Physical activity:** 60% of aging population does not achieve activity recommendations (25% completely inactive); according to data, unfit men who stay unfit increase risk for mortality by less than or equal to 44%; fit individuals, who decrease regular activity over 6 year period increase risk for all-cause mortality by factor of 2; encourage physical activity; important for disease prevention and treatment, prevention of loss of functional abilities, strength, flexibility, elasticity, cardiac and CV function, and for health promotion (even in patients with chronic disease)."[1]

"**Heart Disease:** sedentary population at 2 times higher risk for coronary artery disease than active population; regular physical activity –greater than or equal to 30 min/day of moving body at greater than or equal to 60% maximum capacity (lightly puffing) recommended; aerobic exercise– has beneficial effects on lipids; lowers low-density lipoprotein (LDL); increases high-density lipoprotein (HDL); lowers triglycerides; decreases platelets and fibrin; decreases peripheral vascular resistance by increasing elasticity; sedentary lifestyle – increases risk for cardiovascular disease (CVD) to same degree as having uncontrolled hypertension, smoking one pack of cigarettes per day, or having uncontrolled high cholesterol".[1]

"**Peripheral vascular disease:** improved working capacity seen in older adults who walk, bike, or swim regularly, with higher levels of protective cholesterol and improved lipid ratios."[1]

"**Type 2 diabetes:** relieved by losing weight and exercising (improves carbohydrate metabolism, glycemic control and insulin sensitivity, and reduces secondary complications); rare in individuals with BMI less than 22."[1]

"**Cancer:** good evidence of lower risk for colon cancer in individuals who exercise (may be related to transit time); lower rate of breast cancer seen in fit individuals."[1]

"Depression: talk therapy with exercise found equally as effective as medications (even in schizophrenic and manic depressive patients); aerobic and CV exercise as effective as many forms of psychotherapy and medications; fitness improves mood, irritability, mood swings, self-esteem, and decrease need for psychotropic medications."[1]

"Back pain: exercise for pelvic stability, strength training and postural alignment, and aerobic conditioning can result in less medication use, greater function, lower pain scores, less need for physical therapy, and fewer lost work days."[1]

"Osteoporosis: stressing long bones with axial loading increases bone density; weight- bearing exercise with nutrition, calcium, and vitamin D supplementation important for prevention and minimization of osteoporosis; study – looked at women 60 to 65 years of age; after one year of weight–bearing exercise (greater than or equal to three times per week for 30 minutes), bone density increased by 1.5%, compared to 2.5% loss of bone density in sedentary controls."[1]

"Dementia and AD: physical activity helps brain development; study of rats showed six weeks of exercise (20-30 minutes per day) resulted in 15% increase in synaptic connections; aerobic exercise may be the most powerful predictor of brain neurogenesis (example, creating new effective synaptic connections in brain)."[1]

"Insomnia: study looked at exercise as only treatment in patients 50 to 76 years of age; 30 minutes of exercise per day for 16 weeks reduced time to fall asleep by 50% and increase time asleep by 60 minutes."[1]

"Sarcopenia: at age 50 to 70 years, loss of muscle mass approximately 30% (by age 70 years, 40%; additional 30%

of muscle mass lost every decade after 70 years); resistance training effective in slowing or reversing sarcopenia; quality of lean mass deteriorates unless resistance exercise performed regularly; important to decrease loss of quality lean muscle mass; study–unfit men who became fit had 44% risk reduction in mortality compared to unfit men who remained unfit; decreased physical activity over 6 year period doubled risk of dying."[1]

"Health promotion: important for enjoyment and quality of life; regular exercise reduces stress and symptoms of depression, improves appearance, work capacity, sleep, ability to enjoy leisure time, self-esteem, overall sense of well-being; fitness, flexibility, and closed–chain kinetic activities results in less dyscoordination, less atrophy, less clumsiness, and better range of motion; leads to improved social interactions; exercise shown to influence other healthful choices; study – exercise group 50% more likely to quit smoking, 40% more likely to eat less red meat, 30% more likely to decrease caffeine intake, 250% more likely to eat low-calorie foods, 200% more likely to lose weight, 25% more likely to decrease salt and sugar intake."[1]

"Lifestyle intervention: study – 2006 participants 35 to 65 years of age followed for 8 years; looked at 4 factors (example: smoking, obesity, physical activity [3.5 hours per week], and Mediterranean–type diet); showed 78% reduction in overall chronic disease, 93% risk reduction in diabetes, 81% fewer MIs, 50% fewer strokes, and 36% fewer cancers."[1]

Now you have more information on the dangers of obesity and the benefits of living a healthy lifestyle. So what are you waiting for? Let's get started!

Exercise and Feel Great

Have you ever heard of the expression "Runners High"? This term is used to explain the feeling of overall wellness someone gets after doing strenuous exercise. An example of this would be running three to five miles. In addition to running, you can do other physical activities to get this euphoric feeling: biking, swimming, elliptical, or Stairmaster. A leisurely stroll will probably not get you there. There are many theories as to what causes Runners High. The current theory states that feel good chemicals—endorphins, catecholamine, serotonin, and dopamine—are released by the brain and released into the central nervous system when you do vigorous exercise. [1]

Runners High is thought to be an evolutionary survival mechanism. In the time of early human life, man had to hunt and gather his food to eat and to survive. Early humans had to run long distances to hunt down their food, and it is believed that Runners High was created to prevent them from experiencing pain. Not feeling pain in their legs and feet enabled them to travel long distances, as they hunted their prey.[1]

Some recent studies agree that another neurochemical—endocannabinoids—may cause this euphoric sensation. But regardless of which neurochemical causes Runners High, there is enough evidence to support that it does exist.[1]

Have you ever experienced Runners High? Would you like to? Then let's get moving, so you can experience it! When you do, you will (1) feel better, (2) be encouraged to exercise more often, (3) burn fat, (4) lose weight, and (5) get closer to your ideal goal weight. So get out there, and start to sweat!

Exercise: Get Into a Routine and Stay with It

Losing weight takes determination, along with decreasing the input (what you eat) and increasing the output (the exercise you do). If you were ever an athlete, this is the time to become an athlete again. If you were never an athlete, you need to learn to become one. If you are handicapped, disabled, perhaps missing a limb, or suffering with arthritis or other, you still need to find some way that gets your body moving. Even if you are unable to walk, there are still some physical activities that you can participate in. For example: wheelchair basketball or racing. If you have severe arthritis or chronic pain, water exercises would be the best choice for you: swimming, walking in a pool, or aqua aerobics. The point is to get your body moving. This will help speed up your metabolism, burn fat, and lose weight.

Find a physical activity, sport, or exercise routine you are comfortable with and enjoy doing, and stay with it. I like going to the gym early in the morning and doing one hour of cardiovascular exercise, every day. If you can't go every day, then go six times a week. If you can't go six times a week, then go five times a week. If you can't go five times a week, then go four times a week… You get the idea, right? If you can't or simply don't like going to the gym early in the morning, then go after work or whenever it is best for you. The point is to get into a routine, and repeat it several times a week.

I prefer aerobic exercise versus anaerobic exercise for weight loss. Lifting weights will increase your muscle mass and make you gain weight. You also need to stretch your muscles before and after exercise. I recommend warming up before exercise and cooling down after exercise. This will help to prevent injury.

When you start your weight loss program, start slow and gradually increase. Start by walking twenty minutes, three times a week; then five times a week and then everyday of the week. Once you are comfortable walking 20 minutes a day, increase your time to thirty minutes, three times a week; then thirty minutes, five times a week and again thirty minutes, seven times a week. Your goal should be to walk up to one hour, seven days a week. Once you have conquered this milestone, you are ready to go from walking to jogging. I recommend doing both: walk for five minutes, and jog for five minutes. The goal is to jog the full hour without walking. Some people might not be able to jog. If that is you, try implementing the same escalation of exercise with swimming, biking, tennis, rollerblades, basketball, gliding, rowing, Stairmaster, or other. Whatever exercise you like to do, "Just do it!"

You need to get your metabolism revved up. Your body is like an engine; it needs to burn fuel. What is the fuel? The fuel is the fat inside your body. When you start exercising, you will notice an increase in energy. Your mood will change for the better, and you will begin to feel better overall. However, to successfully accomplish this, you need to choose a routine and stay with it for as long as you can because if you stop your routine, it will be very difficult to start it up again. The only time I recommend stopping a routine is if you get sick or injured. If this happens, you must stop and rest. Once your illness or injury has resolved, you can start to exercise again.

If you exercise, you will lose weight faster, and reach your goal! This is the mentality you must have, at all times. And if you exercise on a regular basis, it will be easier for you to maintain your weight loss. Studies have shown this to be a fact. Exercise *will* decrease your chances of getting obese, Diabetes Mellitus, heart disease, cancer, osteoarthritis/degenerative joint disease, or depression. This is why it is critical to exercise. An extensive global project on disease was conducted, and the conclusion reached was that physical inactivity was one of the biggest risk factors contributing to our decline in health. [1]

If you don't exercise, you will become discouraged because of slow weight loss and frustrating plateaus. The success or failure of this or any other diet and exercise program is up to you and on how serious you are about losing weight.

Variety is key to enjoying and maintaining an exercise program. It will help keep you interested, so you don't get bored. Change up your routine "a little" once in a while. For example, walk on the treadmill for six months, and then switch to the elliptical for six months. During the fall and winter months, the gym is a good place to work out, but in the spring and summer months, exercise outdoors. If you ride your bike for six months, switch and swim for the following six. Another good idea is to use the Stairmaster (or any other machine) for half an hour and then do the other thirty minutes on the elliptical (or another machine). Again, whatever you do, plan for it, and keep going. One last thing, see your doctor before starting a new exercise program.

The Boxers and the Referee

Losing weight and keeping it off is a lifelong battle that we must be determined to win. To help me successfully accomplish this in my own life, I visualized the losing weight process as a boxing match. Yes, losing weight is like a fight or a boxing match. A part of your mind will want to diet and the other part will want to eat. There is also the referee that pushes the two boxers apart. Remember, both fighters will get their punches in and do some damage. This is a battle between fat versus thin. Thin needs to dominate this fight, and win the battle of the bulge. When you implement this diet and exercise program, thin can win. In the past, the fight has gone back and forth. For years, I struggled with this fight, but with this strategy, I have finally defeated the fat fighter and won the championship belt. I am no longer overweight, and I am certain that this diet plan can also help you to win and become a lightweight champion, or whatever weight champion you would like to become. See Chart 1 for men on page 43 and Chart 2 for women on page 44. What is your fighting weight?

Chart 1 - Men

Information from Reference 1

Weight Limit (lib/kg/ Stone)	Con- tinuous since	WA	WBC	IBF	WBO	BoxRec
Unlimited	1885	Heavy weight	Heavyweight	Heavyweight	Heavyweight	Heavyweight
200/90.7/ 14 st 4	1980 [† 1]	Cruiser weight	Cruiser- weight	Cruiser- weight	Junior heavyweight	Cruiser- weight
175/79.4/ 12 st 7	1913	Light Heavyweight	Light Heavyweight	Light Heavyweight	Light Heavyweight	Light Heavyweight
168/76.2/ 12 st	1984	Super middleweight	Super middleweight	Super middleweight	Super middleweight	Super middleweight
160/72.6/ 11 st 6	1884	Middle- weight	Middle- weight	Middle- weight	Middle- weight	Middle- weight
154/69.9/ 11st	1962	Super welterweight	Super welterweight	Junior middleweight	Junior middleweight	Junior middleweight
147/66.7/ 10 st 7	1914	Welter- weight	Welter- weight	Welter- weight	Welter- weight	Welter- weight
140/63.5/ 10 st	1959	Super lightweight	Super lightweight	Junior welterweight	Junior welterweight	Junior welterweight
135/61.2/ 9 st 9	1886	Lightweight	Lightweight	Lightweight	Lightweight	Lightweight
130/59.0/ 9 st 4	1959	Super feath- erweight	Super feath- erweight	Junior lightweight	Junior lightweight	Super feath- erweight
126/57.2/ 9 st	1889	Feather- weight	Feather- weight	Feather- weight	Feather- weight	Feather- weight
122/55.3/ 8 st 10	1976	Super ban- tamweight	Super ban- tamweight	Junior feath- erweight	Junior feath- erweight	Super ban- tamweight
118/53.5/ 8st 6	1894	Bantam- weight	Bantam- weight	Bantam- weight	Bantam- weight	Bantam- weight
115/52.2/ 8 st 3	1980	Super flyweight	Super flyweight	Junior ban- tamweight	Junior ban- tamweight	Super flyweight
112/50.8/ 8 st	1911	Flyweight	Flyweight	Flyweight	Flyweight	Flyweight
108/49.0/ 7 st 10	1975	Light flyweight	Light flyweight	Junior flyweight	Junior flyweight	Light flyweight
105/47.6/ 7 st 7	1987	Minimum- weight	Strawweight	Mini flyweight	Mini flyweight	Minimum- weight

Chart 2 - Women

Information from Reference 1

Professional Women's Weight Divisions
■ Pinweight: up to 101 pounds
■ Light Flyweight: 106
■ Flyweight
■ Light Bantamweight: 114
■ Fetherweight: 132
■ Light Welterweight: 138
■ Welterweight: 145
■ Light Middleweight: 154
■ Middleweight: 165
■ Light Heavyweight: 176
■ Heavyweight: over 189

You Can Still Have Eggs

Eggs are excellent when it comes to weight loss. I used to get upset when I would go on a diet that did not include eggs. Let me explain. Eggs do have a lot of cholesterol and when cooked in butter, the fat content increases exponentially. If eating eggs this way is customary for you, then of course you can't eat eggs while on a diet. However, you *can* eat eggs, and you will eat eggs on this weight loss program. You just have to do it right. Stop using butter! Rather, use a non-stick spray (Pam or Smart Balance non-stick cooking spray). Other ways you can cook the eggs is hard boiled, poached, or microwave them; the latter is a fast and easy way to prepare a fast breakfast because the eggs are done in one minute. Another thing to remember when eating eggs is to limit the intake to one egg per serving. If you need to eat more than one, eat two egg whites. Again, this is all about portion control. Portion control will help eliminate fat, cholesterol, and calories.

Binges and Slip-ups

Everyone will experience moments of weakness when starting a weight loss program, so don't be surprised when you binge or slip-up. Getting angry at yourself over a moment of weakness is not productive. Knowing that these will happen and that there is not much you can do about it will give you clarity of mind to try and keep the damage down to a minimum when it does; if you binge or slip-up, forgive yourself and get back on track with your next meal. When you feel the urge to give in to temptation, here are a few suggestions you can implement to stop the desire to cheat:

- **STOP.** Take a few deep breaths and think about your goals and the progress you have made so far; if you think about this long enough, you might be pleasantly surprised at yourself for having the strength to stop or even to walk away or hold off on the urge to cheat. It will take a few minutes, but the urge will pass.

- **HUNGRY.** You need to get in tune with your stomach. Check to see if you really are hungry. Is your stomach growling? Did you just eat? When was the last time you ate? Trust your stomach, to tell you when it is time to eat.

- **KEEP BUSY.** The best way to avoid binging or cheating is to keep your mind busy with work. If you sit all day watching TV, you are more likely to binge. Doing nothing gives you more time to give in to a few pieces of chocolate or a second slice of pizza. If you must eat the extra food, try to keep the damage to a minimum. If you must cheat, choose to slip-up rather than to have a full blown binge.

- **GET PHYSICAL.** If you can't stop thinking about eating the wrong food, go for a walk, ride your bike, or go to the gym. Any of these activities are much more productive and a lot more fun than taking a trip to the refrigerator.

- **COFFEE OR TEA.** Instead of binging on last night's leftovers, drink a cup of tea or a cup of coffee. A hot cup of coffee with a little bit of skim milk and Truvia (add extra Truvia if your craving for sugar is overwhelming) will suppress your appetite and your cravings fast. This is a great substitute for dessert when you are on a weight loss program.

- **DIET SODA.** If your craving for something sweet feels out of control, a diet soda works well. I don't recommend drinking soda too often. However, drinking one on occasion can help greatly. Diet soda can stop a binge when you are bored. They are also good at parties when everyone else is indulging themselves. When I crave something sweet, they are a good alternative. Remember that I said diet soda—never drink regular soda because they have high sugar content.

- **WATER.** Sometimes a bottle of cool, refreshing water is all you need to suppress your appetite and stop a slip-up or a binge. However, if you need something with flavor, try

"Vitamin Water Zero." (They come in three or four different flavors.) These are delicious, have zero calories, and are full of vitamins, so they are good for you. They are awesome for stopping slip-ups and binges. Again, whatever you do, don't drink the "sugar" variety.

***To help keep you on track** to meet your weight loss goal, you can keep the book in the kitchen while you prepare your meals. You should have a clear view of your diet plan for the day. Prepare each meal as outlined on the diet plan. At the end of the day, look at the list page, and see all the foods that you ate. Use a highlighter marker to highlight the food you ate that day. You should have eaten every food item on the list. Do this every day and every week. It will help you to stay on target to hit your goal.

Also, when you buy your groceries, bring the book with you. You should make a check mark in the box as you take each item off the shelf. When you are ready to pay for your groceries, make sure everything is checked off on the list. This will ensure that you have all the supplies you need for your diet for the week.

There is
Always Monday

Guilt can be our worst enemy when it comes to dieting, so stop feeling guilty if you slip up. Realize that you made a mistake, and get right back on the weight loss program. Make your next meal or snack diet compliant. Plan to eat six small meals a day—about every three to four hours. If you eat this way, you should never feel like you are starving. Pay attention to your stomach signals. It will tell you when it is time to eat—or not eat. Eat each meal as outlined on the plan.

Discipline is important for your short-term and long-term success and following the diet and exercise routine will make it easier to comply. I know you can do it! The fact that you are reading this book lets me know that you are serious about making some positive changes in your life. That's how I know you will succeed. But if in doubt, remember the golden key: will power! We all have it! Do some soul searching and find your will power. Think of it like running a race. If you fall down, you need to get back up, and finish the race. You may not win the race, but you need to cross the finish line. This is not the only race you will participate in, but if you keep practicing, your chances of winning the next race just doubled.

Weekends can be challenging. The temptation to binge may be stronger over the weekend because you might be invited to a party or visit with friends or family where delicious and "irresistible" food will be served. You might drink too much alcohol or enjoy too many sweets. What should you do? Plan for the weekend! Start thinking about what you will eat, ahead of time. Make every effort to stay focused on your weight loss program, but again, if you have a bad eating weekend, don't worry. There is always Monday! Just start all over again [and purpose in your heart to be stronger and to strictly follow the eating program for the week]. This will put you back on track with your weight loss program. Remember, if you make a mistake, if you eat the wrong food, if you slip-up or binge, don't get upset. Start again, right away! It will be a new week. It will be a new start.

A weight loss program is not something we do for a while and then set aside. Eating the right foods and the proper amounts must become a lifestyle. You are about to embark on a new journey of eating and living better. You are finally learning to eat the right way and soon, you will feel great because you will be eating better. You are what you eat. So if you eat garbage, you will feel like garbage, but if you eat healthy, you will feel healthy.

The Basics

It is time to get down to the basics of weight management. The basics set a foundation for success. What are the basics? The basics are protein, carbohydrate, fat, and fiber, in addition to the food pyramid and the input/output formula.

"Protein - Individuals should be counseled to eat a variety of protein rich foods, including fish, lean meat such as poultry, eggs, beans, peas, soy products, and unsalted nuts and seeds. Patients should be advised to avoid protein sources with trans and saturated fats, including red and processed meats. Common sources of dietary protein include whole protein foods (e.g. meat, fish, eggs, vegetables, milk) and protein powders (e.g. casein, whey, soy). The source of protein has a differential effect on health (e.g. red meats are associated with increased mortality, compared to white meats)."[1]

"Carbohydrate – Both the quantity and type of carbohydrate (e.g. simple versus complex, whole grain versus refined grain) have different effects on postprandial glucose levels and glycemic index. Several prospective studies have associated diets high in glycemic index with risk of developing type 2 diabetes mellitus, coronary heart disease, and some cancers. (See Table 1, on page 52, for the Glycemic index of some common foods).

Table 1
Information from reference 1

Dietary glycemic indices and glycemic load for the top 20 Carbohydrate-contributing foods in the Nurses' Health Study in 1984			
Foods	Glycemic Index*, percent	Carbohydrates per serving, g	Glycemic load per serving
Cooked potatoes (mashed or baked)	102	37	38
White bread	100	13	13
Cold breakfast cereal	Varies by cereal	Varies by cereal	Varies by cereal
Dark bread	102	12	12
Orange juice	75	20	15
Banana	88	27	24
White rice	102	45	46
Pizza	86	78	68
Pasta	71	40	28
English muffins	84	26	22
Fruit punch	95	44	42
Cola	90	39	35
Apple	55	21	12
Skim milk	46	11	5
Pancake	119	56	67
Table sugar	84	4	3
Jam	91	13	12
Cranberry juice	105	19	20
French fries	95	35	33
Candy	99	28	28

*Standard reference is white bread, which has a glycemic index of 100%. All other glycemic index values are relative to white bread. *Adapted from: Liu, S. Willett, WC. Dietary glycemic load and atherothrombotic risk. Curr Atheroscler Rep 2002; 4:454*

One important way of achieving a healthy diet is to replace carbohydrates having a high glycemic index (e.g. pizza, rice, pancakes) with a low glycemic index (e.g. fruits, vegetables). Added sugars should comprise no more than 25 percent of total calories consumed."[1]

"**Fat** – The type of fat consumed in a given diet appears to be more important than the amount of total fat (See Table 2, page 54). Saturated fat and Trans fat contribute to coronary heart disease, while monounsaturated and polyunsaturated fats are protective. Individuals should consume less than 10 percent of calories from saturated fatty acids. Saturated fats (e.g. meats, cheese, ice cream) can be replaced with mono-saturated and polyunsaturated fatty acids (e.g. fish, olive oil, and nuts). Patients should be advised to replace fat-full milk products (e.g. whole milk, ice cream) with fat free or low-fat milk products (e.g. skim milk, yogurt, fortified soy beverages). Trans fatty acid consumption should be kept as low as possible. The major sources of Trans fats include margarines and partially hydrogenated vegetable fats. These fats are also present in many processed and fast foods. There is some evidence that long term consumption of fish oil and omega 3 fatty acids reduce the risk of cardiovascular disease. One to two servings of oily fish in the weekly diet is suggested for most adult patients. Consumption of dietary cholesterol should be less than 300mg per day, as recommended by the U.S. dietary guidelines. Consumption of Trans fat, saturated fat, and dietary cholesterol each affect plasma cholesterol levels. Elevated plasma cholesterol concentrations, particularly LDL cholesterol, show a strong and consistent association with the incidence of coronary heart disease (CHD)."[1]

Table 2
Information from reference 1

Sources and main effects of dietary fat				
Type of fat	Chief food sources	Leading food contributors in diets of US adults	Metabolic effects	Effects on disease prevention
TFA, from partiallyhydrogenated vegetables oils	Stick and full fat margarine; commercial baked goods, deep fried foods	Fast food; margarines, baked good (Sweet rolls, cookies, donuts)	Raise LDL – cholesterol. Lower HDL-cholesterol. Raise Lp(a) levels. Interfere with PUFA metabolism	Raise rates of coronary heart disease
SFA	Dairy foods, meat; some plant oils (coconut, palm)	Dairy foods, especially cheese, milk, ice cream; Meat, especially beef, chicken, pork	Raise HDL-C and LDL-C levels; may promote thrombosis	Raise rates of coronary heart disease; may raise risk of prostate, colon cancer
MUFA	Vegetable sources (canola, olive oil); also from meat, dairy, partially hydrogenated oils	Beef; margarines, chicken; olive oil	Lower LDL-C levels slightly Raise HDL-C levels. May interfere with oxidation	Probably lower rates of coronary heart disease
PUFA n-3	For parent alpha-linoleic acid (18.3), an essential FA – canola, soybean, flaxseed, and walnut oil, wheat germ, vegetables of cabbage family For longer chain n-3 FA – seafood, especialy fatty fish	Alpha-linoleic acid (18.3)-mayonnaise, salad dressing, margarines, beef; longer chain n-3 – tuna, other dark rish, shrimp	Is metabolized to longer chain n-3, may decrease thrombosis; important for brain, recinal development; may decrease thrombosis	Increased ratio of n-3: n-6 may decrease rates of coronary heart disease; n-3 may increase birth weight, probably prevent sudden cardiac death
PUFA; n-6	Parent linoleic acid (18:2), an essential FA – many vegetable sources	Mayonnaise; margarines; salad dressing; nuts; chicken; peanut buttter	Arachidonic acid, a metabolite, important in inflammation	Probably reduces rates of coronary heart disease, increased amounts may promote carcinogenesis

Leading food contributors combines the fatty acid content of the food with the frequency with which individuals eat that food. TFA: trans fatty acids; SFA: saturated fatty acids; MUFA: monounsaturated fatty acids; PUFA; polyunsaturated fatty acids. *Data from participants in the ongoing Nurses' Health Study (women) and Health Professional's Follow-up Study (men).

"**Fiber** – The recommended amount of dietary fiber is 14g per 1,000 calories, 25g per day for women and 38g per day for men. Fiber is the portion of plants that cannot be digested by enzymes in the gastrointestinal tract. Fiber is available in a large variety of natural foods and supplements (See Tables 3A, 3B & 3C, pages 57-58). Patients should be advised to replace refined grains (e.g. white rice, white bread) with whole grains (e.g. brown rice, whole wheat bread), which have high fiber content. Increased fiber intake is associated with decreased risk in cardiovascular events and incidence of diabetes—all cause mortality. *Cardiovascular Heart disease:* High fiber intake is associated with a 40 to 50 percent reduction in the risk of CHD and stroke compared with lower fiber intake. A pooled analysis of cohort studies found that each ten gram increase in energy-adjusted intake of fiber per day was associated with a 14 percent relative reduction in the risk for all coronary events and a 27 percent reduction in CHD death. High fiber diets may, in part, protect against CHD by controlling cardiovascular risk factors, including lowering insulin levels, improving lipid profiles, and lowering blood pressure. *Diabetes mellitus*: Fiber consumption from grains also has a protective effect against diabetes mellitus. Increased fiber intake may also be beneficial in controlling blood glucose in patients with established diabetes. *Cancer:* A number of laboratory, nutritional, and epidemiologic studies have identified low levels of dietary fiber in the pathogenesis of colorectal cancer. However, the degree to which dietary fiber protects against the development of adenomas or colorectal cancer is uncertain, since the results of several epidemiologic studies and randomized trials are discordant. *Mortality:* Observational studies suggest that increased dietary fiber intake is associated with decreased all-cause and CHD mortality. In the NIH-AARP cohort, with more than 20,000 male deaths and 10,000 female deaths during nine years of follow up, higher dietary fiber intake was associated with a 22 percent lower risk of all-cause mortality in both men and women (comparing highest to lowest quintiles of fiber intake."[1]

The food pyramid - This chart is a breakdown of the main food groups. This is the absolute basic to being on a diet; the fundamental baseline. Dr. Atkins wrote about turning the triangle upside down. I have tried this, and it does not work for the long term. The best thing to do is to keep it the way it is now. Keep the carbohydrates at the bottom. The next level should be fruits and vegetables. The next level should be dairy, meats poultry, and fish. And at the top of the pyramid are fats, oil, and simple sugar. (See Figure 1 below for full details.)[2]

The input/output formula: This is Diet 101. You need to decrease your input and increase your output. This equals weight loss. If you consume 1,500 calories a day and burn 2,500 calories a day, you will achieve weight loss.

Figure 1 - Food Pyramid
Information from Reference 2

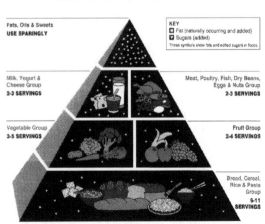

Table 3A *(See page 55)*
Information from reference 1

Provisional Dietary Fiber Table

Food	Fiber, g/serving
Fruits	
Apple (with skin)	3.5/1 medium-sized apple
Apricot (fresh)	1.8/3 apricots
Banana	2.5/1 banana
Cantaloupe	2.7/half edible portion
Dates	13.5/1 cup (chopped)
Grapefruit	1.6/half edible portion
Grapes	2.6/10 grapes
Oranges	2.6/1 orange
Peach	2.1/1 peach
Pear	4.6/1 pear
Pineapple	2.2/1 cup (diced)
Prunes	11.9/11 dried prunes
Raisins	2.2/packet
Strawberries	3.0/1 cup
Juices	
Apple	0.74/1 cup
Grapefruit	1.0/1 cup
Grape	1.3/1 cup
Orange	1.0/1 cup
Vegetables Cooked	
Asparagus	1.5/7 spears
Beans, string, green	3.4/1 cup
Broccoli	5.0/1 stalk
Brussels sprouts	4.6/7-8 sprouts
Cabbage	2.9/1 cup (cooked)
Carrots	4.6/1 cup
Cauliflower	2.1/1 cup
Peas	7.2/1 cup (cooked)
Potato (with skin)	2.3/1 boiled
Spinach	4.1/1 cup (raw)
Squash, summer	3.4/1 cup (cooked, diced)
Sweet potatoes	2.7/1 baked
Zucchini	4.2/1 (cooked, diced)

Reproduced with permission from: The American Gastroenterological Association. Kim YI, Gastroenterology 2000; 118:1235.

Table 3B - Information from reference 1

Provisional dietary fiber table (continued)	
Food	Fiber, g/serving
Raw	
Cucumber	0.2/6-8 slices with skin
Lettuce	2.0/1 wedge iceberg
Mushrooms	0.8/half cup (sliced)
Onions	1.3/1 cup
Peppers, green	1.0/1 pod
Tomatoe	1.8/1 tomatoe
Spinach	8.0/1 cup (chopped)
Legumes	
Baked beans	18.6/1 cup
Dried peas	4.7/half cup (cooked)
Kidney beans	7.4/half cup (cooked)
Lima beans	2.6/half cup (cooked)
Lentils	1.9/half cup (cooked)
Breads, pastas, and flours	
Bagels	1.1/half bagel
Bran muffins	6.3/muffin
Cracked wheat	4.1/slice
Oatmeal	5.3/1 cup
Pumpernickel bread	1.0/slice
White bread	0.55/slice
Whole-wheat bread	1.66/slice

Modified from: the American Gastroenterological Association. Kim YI, Gastroenterology 2000; 118:1235

Table 3C - Information from reference 1

Provisional dietary fiber table (continued)	
Food	Fiber, g/serving
Breads, pastas, and flours (continued)	
Pasta and rice cooked	
Macaroni	1.0/1 cup (cooked)
Rice, brown	2.4/1 cup (cooked)
Rice, polished	0.6/1 cup (cooked)
Spaghetti (regular)	1.0/1 cup (cooked)
Flours and grains	
Bran, oat	8.3/oz
Bran, wheat	12.4/oz
Rolled oats	13.7/1 cup (cooked)
Nuts	
Almonds	3.6/half cup (silvered)
Peanuts	11.7/1 cup

Reproduced with permission from: The American Gastroenterological Association. Kim YI, Gastroenterology 2000; 118:1235.

Table 4 - Information from reference 1

Major food groups	
Grains	Dairy
Whole grains	**Milk**
Brown rice	Fat-free (skim)
Buckwheat	Low-fat (1 percent)
Bulgur (cracked wheat)	Reduced fat (2 percent)
Oatmeal	Whole milk
Popcorn	Flavored milk (eg. Chocolate, strawberry)
Whole grain barley	Lactose reduced milk
Whole grain cornmeal	Lactoce free milk
Whole rye	**Milk-based desserts**
Whole wheat bread	Puddings made with milk
Whole wheat crackers	Ice milk
Whole wheat pasta	Frozen yogurt
Whole wheat sandwich buns and rolls	Ice cream
Whole wheat tortillas	**Cheese**
Wild rice	Cheddar
Less common whole grains	Mozzarella
Amaranth	Swiss
Millet	Parmesan
Quinoa	Ricotta
Sorghum	Cottage cheese
Triticale	American
Ready-to-eat breakfast cereals	**Yogurt**
Whole wheat cereal flakes	Fat-free
Muesli	Low-fat
Refined grains	Reduced fat
Cornbread	Whole milk yogurt
Corn tortillas	**Protein**
Couscous	**Meats**
Crackers	*Lean cuts of:*
Flour tortillas	Beef
Grits	Ham
Noodles	Lamb
White bread	Pork
Whole sandwich buns and rolls	Veal
White rice	Lean luncheon meats
Pitas	*Game meats*
Pretzels	Bison
Pasta	Rabbit
Spaghetti	Venison
Macarroni	*Lean ground meats*
Ready-to-eat breakfast cereals	Beef

Continuation of table 4...

Corn flakes	Pork
Vegetables	Lamb
Artichokes	*Organ meats*
Asparagus	Liver
Bean sprouts	Giblets
Beets	**Poultry**
Brussels sprouts	Chicken
Cabbage	Duck
Cauliflower	Goose
Celery	Turkey
Cucumbers	Ground chicken and turkey
Eggplant	**Eggs**
Green beans	Chicken eggs
Green or red peppers	Duck eggs
Iceberg (head) lettuce	**Dry beans and peas**
Mushrooms	Black beans
Okra	Black-eyed peas
Onions	Chickpeas (garbanzo beans)
Parsnips	Falafel
Tomatoes	Kidney beans
Tomato juice	Lentils
Vegetable juice	Lima beans (mature)
Turnips	Navy beans
Wax beans	Pinto beans
Zucchini	Soy beans
Dark green vegetables	Split peas
Bok choy	Tofu (bean curd made from soy beans)
Broccoli	White beans
Collard greens	*Bean burgets*
Dark green leafy lettuce	Garden burgers
Kale	Veggie burgers
Mesclun	**Nuts and seeds**
Mustard greens	Almonds
Romaine lettuce	Cashews
Spinach	Hazelnuts (filberts)
Turnip greens	Mixed nuts
Watercress	Peanuts
Orange vegetables	Peanut butter
Acorn squash	Pecans
Butternut squash	Pistachios
Carrots	Pumpkin seeds
Hubbard squash	Sesame seeds
Pumpkin	Sunflower seeds
Sweet potatoes	Walnuts

Continuation of table 4...

Starchy vegetables	Fish
Corn	*Finfish such as:*
Green peas	Catfish
Lima beans (green)	Cod
Potatoes	Flounder
Fruits	Haddock
Apples	Halibut
Apricots	Herring
Avocado	Mackerel
Bananas	Pollock
Cherries	Porgy
Grapes	Salmon
kiwi	Sea bass
Mangoes	Snapper
Nectarines	Swordfish
Peaches	Trout
Pears	Tuna
Papaya	*Shelfish such as:*
Pineapple	Clams
Plums	Crab
Prunes	Crayfish
Raisins	lobster
Fruit cocktail	Mussels
Berries	Octopus
Strawberries	Oysters
Blueberries	Scallops
Raspberries	Squid (calamari)
Melons	Shrimp
Cantaloupe	*Canned fish such as:*
Honeydew	Anchovies
Watermelon	Clams
Citrus	Tuna
Grapefruit	Sardines
Lemons	
Limes	
Oranges	
Tangerines	
100 percent fruit juice	
Orange	
Apple	
Grape	
Grapefruit	

Reproduced from: www.mypyramid.gov.

Eating Out
On the Town

When you dine out, the number one rule is: DO NOT EAT THE ROLLS! But if you "must" have a roll, eat only one. You should eat whole wheat or pumpernickel bread instead of white bread. Use olive oil instead of butter. Order a glass of water with a lemon or lime wedge. You can order tea or coffee as well. Order what you want to eat, and split it in half. Share your meal with your spouse, child, or friend, or take the other half home with you. Order a large salad or steamed vegetables as a side dish; this will help fill you up. Skip the dessert, but if you "must" have dessert, order one and split it between three or four people. You should not have more than three to five bites of the dessert. If you add a cup of decaffeinated coffee, with Splenda and skim milk, you should feel completely satisfied. If you are still hungry, take a moment and think about what you will eat for breakfast the next morning. This is an excellent strategy to take when eating out at a restaurant. It works for me all the time.

Filling Up with Fruits and Vegetables

When you eat fruit, eat half. Every morning, you should have a fruit serving for breakfast. For example: half of a banana, half an apple, half a grapefruit, half an orange, or half a cup of grapes, strawberries, prunes, cantaloupe, blueberries, or pineapple. The fruit will help fill you up because they are water dense and full of fiber.

You need to eat vegetables with your lunch and dinner; have as much as you want. These are also water dense and contain plenty of fiber. With lunch, you should have a medium to large salad (use a small amount of low-fat dressing), or you can have broccoli, carrots, green beans, celery sticks, tomato, onion, and cucumber salad. Almost any vegetable will work. But be careful with corn—eating too much of it may slow down weight loss due to its sugar content. If you must have corn, have a small portion without butter. Dinner is the same as lunch. You must add a vegetable serving. Vegetables can be raw, steamed, grilled, or boiled. You can sauté in extra virgin olive oil (small amount). I like to do this with spinach and mushrooms. It makes for an excellent side dish, and it is quite filling.

Eat using a "Volumetrics approach." "Unlike diets based on deprivation, the Volumetrics diet doesn't try to fight this natural preference. Its creator, nutritionist Barbara Rolls, PhD, argues that limiting your diet too severely won't work in the long run. You'll just wind up hungry and unhappy and go back to your old ways."[1]

"Rolls approach is to help people find foods they can eat lots of and still lose weight. The hook of Volumetrics is its focus on satiety—the feeling of fullness. Rolls says that people feel full because of the amount of food they eat, not because of the number of calories or the grams of fat, protein, or carbs. So the trick is to fill up on foods that aren't full of calories. Rolls claims that in some cases, following Volumetrics will allow you to eat more—not less—than you do now, while still slimming down."[1]

Remember to try and change your vegetables at every meal to avoid getting bored with what you eat. Another nice vegetable choice is sliced peppers: red, green, orange, and yellow. They add color and flavor to your plate. If you hate vegetables and there is no way you will eat them, you can substitute the serving of vegetables for 2 servings of any fruit. For example: one apple, one orange, one cup of strawberries, one cup of watermelon chunks, or one cup of grapes. Eating fruit will still allow you to lose weight. Just remember that as a general rule, fruit tends to have more calories than vegetables because of their increased sugar content.

To spice up the flavor of your food, add spices and seasonings, preferably fresh. For example: garlic, oregano, basil, parsley, curry, mustard, and black pepper. Salt, however, should be avoided because it can elevate your blood pressure and make you retain water. Spices and seasonings are important because they have antioxidants and are good for fighting free radicals inside your body. Free radicals can cause cancer, so we need lots of antioxidants to combat them. Other foods that have antioxidants are berries and cinnamon. Try including these in your meals as well.

What is all this talk about free radicals and antioxidants? And what does this have to do with fruits and vegetables? Before I can answer these questions, I need you to think on a cellular level; on a molecular level; on an atomic level; on a subatomic level. In cell death, oxygen is discharged from the cell. This tiny oxygen is known as a free radical;[2] this oxygen is an atom with a positive charge (cation). It is missing an electron. These free radicals can cause a lot of destruction inside the human body, and they have been linked to dementia, heart disease, cancer, and multiple other disease processes.[2] Free radicals circulate in our blood stream wrecking havoc on our healthy tissues, cells and DNA. Antioxidants have a negative charge (anion). They are oxygen atoms with a negative charge. They have an extra electron, so they can bond with the positive charged free radical. Antioxidants bond with the free radicals and stabilize them. Once they are stable, the destruction stops; hence the importance of antioxidants. Once the free radical and antioxidant bond, a stable O_2 molecule is formed.[2] Where do we get antioxidants? Your body can produce antioxidants, but the best way to get them is by eating healthy foods—plant foods—including whole wheat, whole grains, nuts, vegetables, and fruits.[2]

Salad Dressing

No weight loss program can be complete without salad as part of its menu. And no salad will be enjoyed and profitable to the success of the program without the right salad dressing. First thing to consider when it comes to salad dressing is how much to use. Here it is: one tbsp (3 tsp) of light salad dressing is all you need to bring flavor to your salad. The produce section of your local grocery store has a section of low-fat yogurt based salad dressings. There is a wide selection, so choose the ones you like. My particular preference is extra virgin olive oil and rice vinegar. Use only one tablespoon of extra virgin olive oil and as much vinegar as you like. It is very low in calories. Check the calories on the different types of vinegar; they vary. Rice vinegar has about 20 calories per serving, so watch how much you use. Add oregano, basil, garlic powder, and fresh ground pepper for extra flavor. This makes a delicious salad dressing. If you don't like rice vinegar, you can substitute it for balsamic or red wine vinegar—they have fewer calories—or spray on salad dressing.

Salads and salad dressing—type and quantity—play a very important role in the success of this weight loss program. Using too much or the regular calorie salad dressing will add too many calories to your daily food intake and slow down your weight loss. Take your time and taste a variety of low calorie dressings, until you find several that appeal to your taste buds. You want to find a dressing you like so you can enjoy your salad, so select three or four of your favorite low calorie dressings, alternate between them, and enjoy!

Liquids

Water is the best beverage to drink. It is healthy, refreshing, has zero calories, and it gives you a sense of fullness—all of which are essential when it comes to losing weight. Drink lots of water! You need at least 64 oz of water every day (that's eight, 8 oz of water per day); this does not include the coffee, tea, or soda you drink. I suggest drinking 16 oz of water (1 bottle) with each meal—breakfast, lunch, and dinner—and 8 oz with each snack, for a total of 64 oz. This will give you a sense of fullness and suppress your appetite. Of course, drinking this much water will increase your trips to the bathroom, but that's ok because you will definitely be well hydrated.

Water! Water! Water! Push the water. Practice saying to yourself, "Drink the water! Drink the water! Drink the water!" If you practice doing this mentally, you will automatically drink the water. I know it sounds silly, but I actually did this for a while, and it worked!

"Up to 60% of the human body is water. The brain is composed of 70% water, and the lungs are nearly 90% water. Lean muscle tissue contains about 75% water, by weight, as is the brain. Body fat contains 10% water, and bone has 22% water. About 83% of our blood is water, which helps digest our food, transport waste, and control body temperature. Each day, humans must replace 2.4 liters of water, some through drinking and the rest taken by the body from the foods we eat."[1] Since your body is made up mostly of water, you will need to constantly replenish it, especially if you are exercising and sweating. Also, the extra water you drink will help lubricate your bowels, making bowel movement easier.

Want or need flavor in your water? If you don't like plain water and you "must" have some flavor, add a "small" amount of fruit juice. You can drink one fourth of the bottled water and then refill with your favorite fruit juice. That would be one fourth fruit juice and three fourths water. I like to use orange juice, grapefruit juice, apple juice, and cranberry juice. Try to use the no sugar or low sugar alternatives. This will give you less calories for your beverage with that meal. If you use cranberry juice with Splenda, use the formula: one fourth juice with three fourths water. Your beverage will be approximately twenty calories. If you use 4 oz of fruit juice, it will count as one of your fruit servings. You can also do the same thing with sparkling water.

You can add a lemon or lime wedge to add flavor to your water. You can drink it hot or cold. A hot cup of water with lemon in the morning is a great way to start the day. It will help boost your immune system, and it has plenty of antioxidants in the form of vitamin C. My grandfather used to do this every morning, and he lived to be eighty eight years old. It will also help prevent scurvy (a disease caused by a lack of vitamin C). For a refreshing drink on a hot summer day, try zero calorie lemonade. Add three or four lemon wedges to a glass of water and add zero calorie sweetener. Mix the two, add some ice, and there you have it. Drink up and enjoy!

Tea time! You should fill up on green tea, black tea, white tea, and/or herbal tea. There are many varieties to choose from. Tea can be very calming, and it helps to suppress your appetite. You can drink regular or decaffeinated. Green tea is excellent because it has a lot of antioxidants, only a small amount of caffeine to give you a boost during the day, and zero calories. One of my favorite teas is a wellness herbal tea. It contains eucalyptus, Echinacea, vitamin C, and zinc, and you can buy it at your local grocery store. Studies have shown that this combination of ingredients will boost your immune system. This tea is good in preventing the common cold, and it can help get rid of a cold faster. So don't forget your tea time.

Coffee, regular or decaffeinated, can help suppress your appetite. You can have as much coffee as you want on this weight loss program, but do watch the caffeine intake. If your preference is regular coffee, I recommend no more than two cups per day—too much caffeine can cause heart palpitations and blood pressure to elevate.

When drinking tea or coffee, you will want to avoid the cream and sugar. Instead, add 1% or 2% milk, skim or almond milk. Don't use whole milk. Keep in mind that the amount of milk you use in your coffee or tea is "negligible," and it will not slow down your weight loss. Just use small amounts (I add approximately 2 oz to a cup.). If you can drink it plain, it's even better. Sweeten with any sugar substitute; Truvia is a good choice. For a great pick me up or hunger buster drink in the middle of the day or night, drink a large decaffeinated coffee with skim milk and Truvia. You can have it iced or hot. This has saved my diet on several occasions.

Diet soda is fine as a drink, but you will want to keep this down to a minimum because they have a lot of chemicals and are not very healthy, overall. There have been some reports of colas causing cancer. So if you are going to drink soda, try the non-cola versions, and watch the caffeine intake here as well.

Use extreme caution when it comes to alcohol because it will slow down your weight loss. I recommend not drinking alcohol while on this weight loss program. However, if you simply can't do without it, I recommend saving it for the weekend or for special occasions. Red wine has a lot of antioxidants and is good for the cardiovascular system. Rosa and white wine are also good but not as good as red wine. Red wine is the best choice because the skin of the grape contains a chemical called "resveratrol" which has proven cardiovascular protection.[2] In my opinion, the best red wine choice to drink is the Merlot followed by the Cabernet. If beer is your alcohol of choice, light beer—preferably ultra-light—is the way to go. I don't recommend hard liquor. However, if you choose to indulge, be careful what you mix it with. Men should not have more than two alcoholic beverages per day/night and women no more than one per day/night. Remember, the key to the success of this weight loss program is portion control. Warning: drinking alcohol weakens your inhibitions, and you will most likely eat and drink more and be at risk for slip ups and binges.

Other drinks allowable include: Vitamin water Zero (as discussed in an earlier chapter); tomato juice, the low sodium version, as much as you like; a cup of skim milk every morning and evening. Skim milk usually has vitamins A and D added. One serving size has approximately ninety calories, zero fat, thirteen grams of carbohydrate, and nine grams of protein. Almond milk is currently my favorite beverage, as it contains thirty or forty calories, 3.5 grams of fat (zero saturated fat), two grams of carbohydrate, and one gram of protein. Flax seed milk is a new discovery of mine. It is about 50 calories per serving, and it is full of omega three—this means it is cardiac protective and great if you suffer from constipation as it helps stimulate bowel movements. All you need is half a cup. Soy slender is a soy based, non-dairy beverage and sweetened with Splenda. You can substitute your milk serving with Soy slender. It comes in three different flavors: vanilla, chocolate, and cappuccino.

Hot soup or broth will help control and suppress your appetite. Have one cup before a meal, when desired. Good choice soups are: vegetable soup, tomato soup, or chicken broth. Cold soup is also good; try gazpacho soup.

Your Plate

When serving your meal (this mostly applies to lunch and dinner), use smaller sized plates, rather than large plates, for better portion control. Divide it into three sections; think of this image in your mind (See figure 2 below). This is a very simple concept, and it works great to keep you on target for your weight loss goal. Now, look at the palm of your hand. That is the size portion of the protein that you want to eat; approximately four 4 oz. The complex carbohydrate portion should be no bigger than a tennis ball or a baseball; approximately half a cup to one full cup of, for example, rice, potato, pasta, or one slice of bread. The remainder of your plate should be all vegetables. In other words, one quarter of the plate protein, one quarter of the plate complex carbohydrate, and half a plate of vegetables.[1] If you can't stand vegetables, you can replace them with fruit. For example, one apple instead of a salad with dressing.

Figure 2 - Your Plate

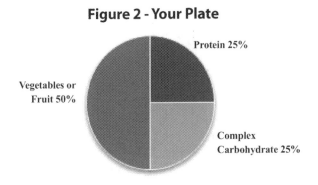

Get in the Zone

What is "the zone"? Do you remember when Michael Jordan was on fire, hitting all his shots when playing basketball for the Chicago Bulls? He was dominating the basketball world! Or Eli Manning of the New York Giants who made every play in the fourth quarter, by the end of the 2011–2012 football season, and later went on to win the Super Bowl? And Lebron James of the Miami Heat winning his first NBA championship and now trying to win multiple championships and create a dynasty. That is the answer to the question: "What is the zone?" This phrase describes athletes when they just can't do anything wrong. The basketball rim looks like the size of a hula hoop, or a baseball is the size of a melon. The athlete is in the zone. Well, you need to get into the diet zone.

How do you get in the zone? You start by eating those six small meals, perfectly portioned with the right combination of carbohydrate, protein, fat, and fiber; by exercising every day for one hour and working up a good sweat. In the zone, you will feel amazing and have great energy. You will be firing on all cylinders, and the pounds will start coming off you every week. When you establish a routine and stick to your program, you will enter the zone and stay there. And before you know it, you will have reached your goal. If you eat this way and exercise regularly, you will perform better at work and in school. If you are an athlete, you will perform better in athletic competition.

Think and Lose Weight

You need to constantly think about making the right decisions while on this weight loss program. You might not always make the right choices, but you will need to strive for 90% of the time. If you think and plan out all your meals, you will be successful in your weight loss goals. On this program, you will need to go to the grocery store at least once a week to keep your pantry filled with your favorite diet food items. This will help make your decisions easier. My family likes to go out for brunch often; usually for special occasions or holidays. This can be a challenge because there is always an abundance of food and plenty of opportunities to surrender to temptation. When occasions like this come up, you need to think in advance about what you are going to eat, and plan to stay with that thought. Do not deviate from your plan. Think of a strategy that will keep you diet compliant. The holidays can also be challenging, but again, plan in advance. Try and stay as close as you can to your diet regiment. If you deviate a little, it's OK! as long as you get right back on your diet program after the weekend or the holiday. Remember, you want to minimize the damage as much as possible—practice damage control.

Focus on the food while you are eating. Remember, this is where you get your energy from. Your portions will be smaller than before you started the diet, so make sure you chew your food slowly and completely. Sit down to eat. Never eat standing up. Eat on a comfortable chair in a well lit room, so you can see what you are eating and enjoy it. Do not watch TV while eating because it takes your focus away from your food.

Pay attention to your stomach. It will tell you when it is time to eat. On this diet, you will be eating small meals every three to four hours. However, you still need to be aware of your stomach signals. When you eat, pay attention to how full you feel. Are you empty (starving), half full, full, half over full, or stuffed? Try to stay in the full range after eating (satisfied). Take the time to think how you feel after eating. If you get too hungry, you will have a tendency to overeat and go off your diet. So make sure you eat all six, small frequent meals. That way you should never feel like you are starving. Think before you eat, and make sure the portions are right. Now go ahead and enjoy your meal!

Attack Obesity from Three Directions: Diet, Exercise, and Brain Power

This is not a complicated diet to follow. All you have to do is eat the foods on the schedule, and you will lose weight. Get into an exercise routine, and stay with it. Remember to try and go every day for one hour. Start slow and gradually increase your frequency and duration of time. Brain power is important because you need to think and make the right decisions. If you use all three components: diet, exercise, and brain power, you can defeat obesity.

Dessert and Chocolate

Dessert is very important. I want you to reward yourself every night with a good, healthy dessert. Again, the portions must be small, and you should have dessert with some type of milk (I like to use almond milk because it has the perfect blend of protein, carbohydrate, and good fat.). One cup of milk with your small dessert is the perfect combination. If you prefer skim, soy, rice, or flaxseed milk, keep in mind that they have more calories per cup, and if you chose almond milk, I recommend the sugar free variety. You can always add some sweetener to satisfy your sweet tooth. If you go out for dessert, you should split or share. Some of my favorite desert options are low-fat ice cream or low-fat frozen yogurt on a stick. These desserts are already portioned out for you. You can add one glass of almond milk (chocolate or vanilla) for an additional 40 calories. Try to avoid the ice cream in the half gallon containers because it makes it difficult to control portion size. I love ice cream and can easily enjoy a whole cup instead of a ½ cup. For me this is difficult to control, so I recommend not buying the ½ gallon containers; only the portioned out, low-fat, low sugar variety. Never get full fat ice cream. Fresh fruit with 6 oz of nonfat or low-fat yogurt is an excellent alternative.

One serving of low-fat cookies and a cup of almond milk is also a great choice. This will satisfy your need for sweets. Another great dessert is two cups of almond milk, two packs of Truvia, and some nonfat or low-fat whip cream on top; this dessert tastes great, like a milkshake, and it has less than 100 calories, and it really fills you up.

Chocolate? Yes! You can have chocolate. Almond and Soy milk both come in chocolate flavor. Chocolate almond milk is only forty five calories. If you combine two cups, you have a ninety calorie chocolate beverage. This is a delicious desert that will satisfy any chocoholic. You can drink this any time of the day. Dark chocolate is an excellent alternative to the more fatty milk chocolate. It is lower in fat and sugar content, and it is loaded with antioxidants. One ounce of dark chocolate for dessert, with milk, and you are good to go! You can use Weight Watchers chocolate desserts on this diet. I have incorporated both Weight Watchers brownies and Weight Watchers chocolate ice cream bars into this diet. They are excellent and can be purchased in your local grocery store. A Kashi brownie is another good option. So you see, you have several options for desserts, as long as you practice portion control.

Get a Support Group

Everyone needs support when starting a weight loss program. It is very difficult to do it on your own. Ask a friend or your significant other to participate on the diet with you, or you can make this a family—children included—affair. They can help you shop for the food and help prepare your meals. Dieting with others will make the process less difficult and it offers the support you need to persevere. It is good to have someone to share how your day went with your diet; someone to motivate you; someone to encourage you if you slip up; someone to exercise with you, and when you reach your goal, someone to celebrate with. Your partner can help push you when it becomes difficult. And they will not let you quit until you reach your goal. If you don't live with the person, your partner is only a phone call away.

It would also be a good idea to consult with a professional—a doctor, a dietician, a nutritionist and/or a personal trainer. The key thing here is to realize the importance of a support group.

Body Mass Index (BMI)

What is BMI? "Body mass index is defined as the individual's body weight divided by the square of his or her height. The formula universally used in medicine produce a unit of measure of KG/m2. BMI can also be determined using a BMI chart, which displays BMI as a function of weight (horizontal axis) and height (vertical axis) using contour lines for different values of BMI or colors for different BMI categories (See Formula 1 below, and Graph 1 on pg. 82)"[1] Also see Chart 1 on pg. 83 and determine your BMI. This will give you a good idea of what your goal weight should be. Your goal weight should be found in the normal BMI range.

Formula 1

Information from reference 1

SI units	$BMI =$	$\dfrac{\text{mass (kg)}}{(\text{height (m)})^2}$
Imperil/US Customary Units	$BMI =$	$\dfrac{\text{mass (lb) x 703}}{(\text{height (in)})^2}$
	$BMI =$	$\dfrac{\text{Mass (lb) x 4.88}}{(\text{height) (ft)})^2}$

Graph 1
Weight [pounds]
Information from reference 1

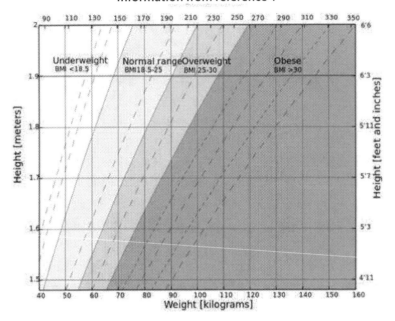

A graph of body mass index as a function of body mass and body height is shown above. The dashed lines represent subdivisions within a major class. For instance the "Underweight" classification is further divided into "severe", "moderate", and "mild" subclasses.1

Chart 1
Information from Reference 2

BMI	21	22	23	24	25	26	27	28	29	30	35	40	41	42
Height (in.)	Weight (lb.)													
58	100	105	110	115	119	124	129	134	138	143	167	191	196	201
59	104	109	114	119	124	128	133	138	143	148	173	198	203	208
60	107	112	118	123	128	133	138	143	148	153	179	204	209	215
61	111	116	122	127	132	137	143	148	153	158	185	211	217	222
62	115	120	126	131	136	142	147	153	158	164	191	218	224	229
63	118	124	130	135	141	146	152	158	163	169	197	225	231	237
64	122	128	134	140	145	151	157	163	169	174	204	232	238	244
65	126	132	138	144	150	156	162	168	174	180	210	240	246	252
66	130	136	142	148	155	161	167	173	179	186	216	247	253	260
67	134	140	146	153	159	166	172	178	185	191	223	255	261	268
68	138	144	151	158	164	171	177	184	190	197	230	262	269	276
69	142	149	155	162	169	176	182	189	196	203	236	270	277	284
70	146	153	160	167	174	181	188	195	202	207	243	278	285	292
71	150	157	165	172	179	186	193	200	208	215	250	286	293	301
72	154	162	169	177	184	191	199	206	213	221	258	294	302	309
73	159	166	174	182	189	197	204	212	219	227	265	302	310	318
74	163	171	179	186	194	202	210	218	225	233	272	311	319	326
75	168	176	184	192	200	208	216	224	232	240	279	319	327	335
76	172	180	189	197	205	213	221	230	238	246	287	328	336	344

BMI CHART KEY: *Normal:* 18-24 **Overweight:** 25-29 **Obese** 30-39 *Extremely obese:* 40 and above. /find an expanded BMI table at www.nhlbi.nih.gove/guidelines/obesity/bmi_tbl.pdf

Glycemic Index

"The Glycemic Index or GI is a measure of the effects of carbohydrates on blood sugar levels. Carbohydrates that break down quickly during digestion and release glucose rapidly into the blood stream have a high GI; carbohydrates that break down slowly and release glucose gradually into the blood stream, have a low GI. The concept was developed by Dr. David J. Jenkins and colleagues in 1980-1981, at the University of Toronto, in the research to find out which foods were best for people with diabetes. A lower glycemic index suggests slower rate of digestion and absorption of the food's carbohydrates and may also indicate greater extraction from the liver periphery of the products of carbohydrate digestion. A lower glycemic response usually equates to a lower insulin demand, but not always, and may improve long-term blood glucose control and blood lipids."[1]

What does all this mean in laymen's terms? A food that is high on the GI scale would be white bread (100), and a food that is low on the GI scale would be an apple (55). When you eat a piece of white bread, it goes into the stomach and is rapidly absorbed into the blood stream. At that point in time, a lot of insulin is secreted to transport the glucose into your cells. When you eat an apple, it takes longer to digest. This is mostly due to the fiber content of the apple. It will take time, and the glucose enters the blood stream slowly. Also, insulin will be released at a slower rate. This is important because it will prevent your blood glucose levels from going too high or too low, and this helps to stabilize your cravings for food.

So the foods you want to avoid are the ones that are high on the glycemic index scale. For example: white bread, white rice, and corn flakes. The foods you want to eat a lot of are low on the glycemic index scale. For example: skim milk, apples, and celery (see table 5 below).

Table 5
Information from reference 1

Classification	GI range	Examples
Low GI	55 or less	Most fruits and vegetables, legumes/pulses, some whole, intact grains, nuts, fructose
Medium GI	56-69	Whole wheat products, basmati rice, sweet potato, sucrose, baked potatoes
High GI	70 and above	White bread, most white rices, corn flakes, extruded breakfast cereals, glucose, maltose, maltodextrins

Vitamins and Medication

The only vitamin you will need on this diet is one: I like to use "Centrum Performance." It has ginkgo biloba and ginseng added to the multivitamin. Ginkgo biloba is good to increase your memory, and ginseng will increase your energy level. This should help keep you on track with the foods you should eat and your exercise routine. If you are over sixty, Centrum silver is a good choice. No other vitamins are needed on this diet.

Medicine that can help you lose weight includes:

1. Antidepressants; Wellbutrin will suppress the appetite by increasing dopamine and norepinephrine in your brain and cause your body's metabolism to increase. The problem with this medicine is that it causes your blood pressure and heart rate to elevate.[1]

2. Other antidepressants that may help you lose weight are SSRI's. Examples of these are Paxil and Zoloft. Sometimes, they are used in combination with Wellbutrin. It increases serotonin in your brain and are classified as anti-depressants.[1]

3. Medicine that affects GABA (gamma-amino-butyric acid). Topamax is a drug that decreases the nerve activity from your brain to your gut. This will decrease your desire to eat. One of the side effects is sedation.[1]

4. Xenical and Alli block the absorption of fat. You can lose up to 10% of your body weight on these medications.[1] Side effects include fecal incontinence if you eat too much fat. Be very careful not to eat a lot of fat if you take this medicine.

5. Glucophage can help decrease weight by making the insulin inside your body more effective. Glucose will go back to normal levels because insulin is working more efficient and Insulin will help transport the glucose back inside the cell (the glucose will get metabolized inside the cell).[1]

6. Precose is also used to help with weight loss. This medication blocks absorption of sugar. Side effects include flatus and diarrhea.[2]

7. Adipex –P (Phentermine) is a sympathomimetic.[2] This drug increases metabolism and decreases appetite. Side effects include CNS over stimulation, palpitations, hypertension and cardiac arrhythmias.[2] This medication must be taken early in the day.[2] You don't want to take it before bedtime. I recommend having a complete blood test before starting this medication. This would include a complete blood count, complete metabolic profile, thyroid stimulating hormone, liver function tests, and an electrocardiogram.

Also check the BMI. This should be "greater than or equal to 30Kg/m2 or greater than or equal to 27Kg/m2" if other co-morbidities exist.[2]

8. Caffeine and nicotine can also be used to suppress your appetite. Caffeine in coffee or tea works well. I don't recommend nicotine for weight loss.

Maintaining Your Weight Loss

Once you reach your goal weight, you will maintain it by adding a few hundred calories to your daily food intake. This can be done by adding a slice of wheat bread to your lunch or dinner or both. You can have a glass of wine or light beer with dinner or add an extra half cup of brown rice, sweet potato, or multigrain pasta to your lunch/dinner or both. You can also add some extra protein to your meal. For example an extra egg white, 2-4 ounces of sliced turkey breast, salmon or chicken. Start by doing this three times a week; then increase it to five times a week. Weight yourself once a week. If you go five pounds over your goal weight, return to the weight loss program.

Instead of increasing your food intake, you can decrease your exercise program—but only a little. For example, instead of exercising every day, you can do it three times per week. All you have to remember is the input, output formula. If the calories you intake are the same as the calories you burn, you will maintain your weight. You will maintain your weight if you continue to eat six small meals a day and simply add a few extra calories—approximately 200 to 300 more calories per day and you should stabilize.

Looking at Labels

Get used to reading food labels. This is a very important habit to get into to gain awareness of your food intake. You will want to check the saturated fat content in a food, and if it is greater than three, don't eat it. Check for calories, fiber, and sodium. You want high fiber, low sodium, and low sugar content. Polyunsaturated fat and monounsaturated fat are OK to eat. Try to keep high fructose corn syrup down to a minimum. Avoid all hydrogenated and partially hydrogenated fats and anything with food coloring. If there are too many chemicals listed on the label, don't eat that food item. Try to eat non processed foods. I know this is hard to do but try anyway.

You want to eat whole foods. The best snacks come unwrapped; for example, fruits and nuts. On this diet, you can eat a variety of foods. It is just more simple, convenient, and practical that way. You can fine tune your diet once you reach your weight loss goal. The main goal right now is to get you to lose weight. On this diet, there are small amounts of chips, cookies and other wrapped items that you will enjoy eating. This diet is meant to reach a lot of different people. If you want, you can replace the chips and cookies with other whole foods such as fruits, vegetables, and nuts. "It's now known that trans fat is a major contributor (along with saturated fat) to coronary heart disease."[1]

Favorite Cheats and Still Be Diet Compliant

It is extremely difficult to successfully complete a weight loss program if we are forced to give up all the foods we enjoy. On this program, you will be able to enjoy great food from some of your favorite places. For example:

Breakfast: <u>McDonalds</u> — Egg McMuffin, 1 side of fruit and yogurt, 1 lowfat milk and coffee. <u>Dunkin Donuts</u> — 1 glazed donut, bring your own fruit, ½ coffee and ½ skim milk (get the large size); or a bran muffin or low-fat blueberry muffin (eat only half), bring your own fruit, ½ coffee and ½ skim milk.

Lunch: <u>Char Hut</u> — 1 grilled chicken or tuna on a whole wheat bun with vegetables and a small side of hot sauce; add a large garden salad with light salad dressing and a bottle of water. <u>Mo's Bagel and Deli</u> — tuna salad on whole wheat bagel with lettuce tomato and onion; only eat half of the sandwich. Add a small vegetable soup, and drink only half, plus a bottle of water. <u>Subway</u> — six inch veggie sub, baked potato chips, plus one bottle of water.

Dinner: If you eat out, spilt the meal with your significant other, your child, or a friend. Order a side of vegetables or a salad for each person sharing the meal.

Dessert: <u>TCBY</u> is always a good choice — a small low-fat frozen yogurt (Golden Vanilla is my personal favorite), and top it off with almonds. <u>Dairy Queen</u> — one small soft serve in a cup or a sugar-free Dilly Bar. Enjoy your dessert but be careful not to cause serious damage to your weight loss program (remember: damage control).

Miscellaneous: Avoid all fast food restaurants as best you can. That includes fast food burger restaurants and fried chicken restaurants. Avoid what I call Danger Zone Restaurants. This is where you can do serious damage to your diet program. If you know you cannot control yourself there, don't go there. These include but are not limited to Chinese buffets, brunch buffets, cruise buffets, and favorite dessert restaurants. Stay out of the danger zone. When going to the movies, bring your own snacks.

Emergency Foods

When you are starving and you know you have to eat, reach for your emergency foods. You can eat any fruit, one cup extra per day to control hunger—and as much vegetables as you want. Good examples are: apples, celery stalks, cucumber, or carrot sticks. I like to use sautéed spinach in light olive oil with added seasoning (no salt). In an emergency, drink as much V-8 tomato juice (the low sodium variety) as you like. In an emergency, you can also have extra lean protein (sliced turkey breast is a good choice) or coffee, as previously discussed.

Condiments

No one likes to eat bland, flavorless foods. A good weight loss program requires good food to eat so I recommend the basics: ketchup, mustard, light mayonnaise, barbeque sauce, salsa, Worcestershire sauce, teriyaki sauce, low sodium soy sauce, steak sauce, and tomato sauce (½ a cup is 1 serving). Keep track of the calories and serving sizes. You should need no more than one serving size of these items.

Sweeteners

It's all about flavor. It is hard to be faithful to a weight loss program when the foods we eat have no taste. Some experts recommend not using sweeteners—sugar substitutes—but I have tried this, and it is almost impossible for me. I use sweeteners in a lot of different things including coffee, tea, and oatmeal. Some diet products don't need additional sweeteners because they already have it as part of their ingredients. My personal favorite is Truvia; it looks and tastes like sugar. Other sweeteners are: Sweet and Low (saccharine), NutraSweet (aspartame), Splenda (sucralose), and Stevia. Choose the one you like best, or don't use any at all. Saccharine has been around the longest. They have a warning sign on the label stating that use of the product may cause cancer. However, studies were not done on humans, and one must consume huge quantities of the product for this to happen. The next sweetener to enter the market was NutraSweet, followed by Splenda. More studies need to be done to see the long term effects of these sugar substitutes on the human body. Stevia was next to enter the market. This product comes from a plant; it is all natural. However, this product tends to have an after taste. The newest product is Truvia. This product tastes and its texture is very similar to table sugar, and it has zero calories.

Other sweeteners that can be used are honey, agave nectar, brown sugar, and white refined sugar (table sugar). If you use any of these products, use them sparingly. They tend to have a lot of calories and will slow weight loss. Honey is all natural, and it has no preservatives. Agave nectar is very sweet, and you only need a small amount. This product is also all natural; no preservatives. Brown sugar is all natural and has no preservatives. I tend to use this when there is no better alternative. I use table sugar only as a last resort.

Recipes

GOOD MORNING SANDWICH

    1 egg (can substitute with 2 egg whites)
    1 multigrain English muffin
    1 slice low-fat cheese
    1 pinch fresh ground pepper
    ½ oz ketchup or salsa

Spray medium size frying pan with nonstick spray and cook egg as desired. Place cooked egg on toasted English muffin, add cheese, and top with pepper and ketchup or salsa. (1 serving)

ONE MINUTE EGG SANDWICH

    1 egg (can substitute with 2 egg whites)
    1 slice whole wheat toast
    1 tsp low-fat shredded cheddar cheese
    1 tsp chopped onion
    1 pinch ground pepper
    ½ oz ketchup

Spray small bowl with non-stick spray. Add egg and scramble. Mix in onion, black pepper and cheddar cheese.

Cook in microwave for 1 minute. Cut the whole wheat toast in half and place the cooked egg on it. Top with ketchup and with the other ½ slice of toast.

CINNAMON FRENCH TOAST (2 Servings)

4 eggs
3 slices whole wheat bread
¼ to ½ tbsp cinnamon
1 oz light maple syrup

Scramble eggs in a large bowl. Add the cinnamon as you mix. Spray a medium frying pan with non stick spray and place on medium heat. Dunk the bread in egg mixture and fry in the pan. Cook both sides well. Serve one and a half slice of French toast and top with maple syrup. (2 servings)

TUNA AND TOMATO WHEEL

1 can albacore white tuna
1 tbsp light mayonnaise
1 slice chopped onion
1 thick slice of tomato
1 celery stalk chopped
1 slice whole wheat bread
1 dash fresh black pepper
1 dash oregano
1 dash basil
1 dash garlic powder

Combine all ingredients in a large bowl. Toast the bread. Place 2 tbsp of tuna salad on top of the toast, add the tomato slice, and enjoy. (1 serving)

TOMATO, ONION, AND CUCUMBER SALAD

1 ripe tomato
¼ cup chopped onion
½ cucumber peeled and sliced
1 dash oregano
1 dash basil
1 dash garlic powder
1 dash black pepper
1 tbsp extra virgin olive oil
3 tbsp rice vinegar or balsamic vinegar

Mix all ingredients in large bowl and enjoy. (1 serving)

CHICKEN SALAD

1 chicken breast grilled or baked then cubed
1 tbsp light mayonnaise
1 slice chopped onion
½ apple chopped
1 celery stalk chopped

Combine all ingredients in a large bowl and serve. (2 servings)

CHICKEN FAJITAS

1 chicken breast
½ sliced onion cut into small pieces
1 red pepper
1 green pepper
4 whole wheat tortillas
½ cup light cheese

½ cup light sour cream
½ cup salsa
½ cup guacamole

Spray medium size pan with nonstick spray and heat on medium high. Sautee peppers and onion for five minutes. Remove and place in small bowl. Re-spray pan and grill chicken breast until done; slice into strips. Place 1 heated tortilla on a plate and place 2 chicken strips, 1 red pepper strip, 1 green pepper strip, 2 to 3 onion strips, 1 tsp of cheese, 1 tsp of sour cream, 1 tsp of salsa, and 1 tsp of guacamole. Fold tortilla and enjoy. This recipe makes 4 fajitas. (2 servings)

FRIED CHICKEN WITH SEASONED BREAD CRUMBS

2 chicken breasts
3 eggs
1 cup seasoned bread crumbs
1-2 tbsp of extra virgin olive oil

Trim the fat off the chicken breast and cut in half. Dip in egg and then in seasoned bread crumbs. Coat medium to large pan with olive oil and discard the excess oil; heat on medium high. Turn heat down to medium and add chicken. Cook both sides until golden brown. Cover with lid to decrease cooking time. (4 servings)

FRIED TALAPIA WITH SEASONED BREAD CRUMBS

2 8 oz tilapia
3 eggs
1 cup seasoned bread crumbs
1-2 tbsp of extra virgin olive oil

Dip tilapia in egg and bread crumbs. Coat medium to large pan with olive oil and discard the excess oil; heat on medium high. Turn heat down to medium and add tilapia. Cook both sides until golden brown. Cover with lid to decrease cooking time. (4 servings)

CHICKEN PARMESAN

2 chicken breasts
3 eggs
1 cup seasoned bread crumbs
½ cup tomato sauce
4 oz mozzarella cheese

Preheat oven to 425 degrees. Clean chicken breast, trim fat, and cut in half. Dip in egg and toss in bread crumbs. Place chicken in baking pan. Bake for 25 minutes. Add tomato sauce and sprinkle 1 oz of cheese on top of chicken and bake for 5 additional minutes. Remove from oven and serve. (4 servings)

EGG SALAD

1 hardboiled egg
1 tsp of light mayonnaise
1 tsp chopped onion
1 tsp chopped celery
1 pinch black pepper
1 pinch garlic powder

Chop eggs and combine all ingredients. (1 serving)

Quick Dessert Recipes

100 CALORIE MILKSHAKE

Chocolate or vanilla almond milk, unsweetened and chilled

   2 tbsp low-fat or nonfat light whip cream

   2-4 packets of Truvia (to sweeten to taste)

Shake almond milk well. Pour 16 oz into a glass and add Truvia to taste. Top off with whip cream.

200 CALORIE MILKSHAKE

Chocolate or vanilla almond milk, unsweetened and chilled

   2 tbsp low-fat or nonfat light whip cream

   2-4 packets of Truvia (to sweeten to taste)

   ½ ripe banana

Pour 16 oz of almond milk into blender; add banana, Truvia to taste, blend, and serve.

Top off with whip cream.

300 CALORIE MILKSHAKE

Chocolate or vanilla almond milk, unsweetened and chilled

2 tbsp low-fat or nonfat light whip cream

2-4 packets of Truvia

½ ripe banana

½ cup low-fat frozen yogurt, vanilla, or chocolate

Pour 16 oz of almond milk into blender; add banana, Truvia to taste, frozen yogurt, and blend. Serve and top off with whip cream.

The 8 Week Plan

Week 1

GROCERY LIST

Always have the following on hand:

- ☐ Bottles of water (16.9 FL OZ - 24 pack).
- ☐ Water (1 gallon - purified)
- ☐ Coffee
- ☐ Green tea
- ☐ Light salad dressing
- ☐ Rice vinegar or Balsamic
- ☐ Nonstick spray
- ☐ Extra virgin olive oil
- ☐ Light cranberry juice
- ☐ Ground flaxseeds (organic)
- ☐ Cinnamon
- ☐ Fresh black pepper
- ☐ Garlic powder
- ☐ Basil
- ☐ Oregano
- ☐ Mustard
- ☐ BBQ sauce
- ☐ Ketchup

- ☐ Light mayonnaise
- ☐ Organic honey
- ☐ Truvia (or sweetener of choice)
- ☐ Aluminum foil
- ☐ Small, medium, and large size reusable plastic containers

....

- ☐ Eggs (organic brown)
- ☐ Low-fat cheese ¼ lb
- ☐ Milk (skim, soy, almond, or flaxseed)
- ☐ Yogurt (5 nonfat 6 oz)

- ☐ Brown rice
- ☐ Kashi cereal Go Lean Crunch
- ☐ Multigrain pasta
- ☐ Quaker Oatmeal (not the instant type)
- ☐ Whole wheat buns
- ☐ Whole wheat double fiber bread

- ☐ Apples (organic)
- ☐ Bananas
- ☐ Grapes
- ☐ Grapefruits (may substitute with other fruit)

- ☐ 1 potato or sweet potato
- ☐ Baby carrots
- ☐ Broccoli
- ☐ Celery sticks
- ☐ Corn on the cob

- ☐ Cucumber (1)
- ☐ Green beans (2 packages)
- ☐ Mixed vegetables
- ☐ Sweet onion (1)
- ☐ Romaine lettuce (2 packages)
- ☐ Tomatoes (4)

- ☐ Albacore tuna (1 can)
- ☐ Baked beans (fresh from favorite BBQ restaurant)
- ☐ Beef (lean)
- ☐ Chicken breast
- ☐ Chicken noodle soup (buy from deli or restaurant)
- ☐ Salmon
- ☐ Turkey breast (¼ lb sliced)
- ☐ Turkey burgers (extra lean)

- ☐ Chips Ahoy reduced fat cookies
- ☐ Eddy's frozen coconut bars (may substitute with other frozen fruit bars)
- ☐ Jala bars (frozen low-fat yogurt)
- ☐ Kashi Chewy Granola Bars
- ☐ Roasted almonds (no salt)
- ☐ Smart'n Healthy popcorn

- ☐ 1 jar tomato sauce
- ☐ Light maple syrup
- ☐ Salsa
- ☐ Smucker's organic peanut butter

WEEK 1 DAY 1

BREAKFAST

2 egg whites (fry in pan using nonstick spray)
1 slice whole wheat toast
1 fruit serving (examples ½ banana, ½ apple, ½ grapefruit or ½ orange)
1 cup milk (may substitute with soy, almond, or flaxseed milk)
1 cup of coffee or tea
1 cup of water

SNACK

1 Kashi Bar
1 cup water

LUNCH

2 slices turkey breast on 1 slice whole wheat bread
1 tbsp mustard, ketchup, or light mayonnaise
Green tea
1 bottle of water

SNACK

10 roasted almonds
1 cup water

DINNER

4 oz chicken breast (baked)
½ cup brown rice
½ plate steamed mixed vegetables
1 bottle water

DESSERT

1 Eddy's frozen coconut bar (may substitute with other frozen fruit bar)
1 cup skim milk (may substitute with soy, almond, or flaxseed milk)

WEEK 1 DAY 2

BREAKFAST
½ cup oatmeal (cook in 1 cup of water)
Truvia or choice of sweetener and sprinkle with 1 tsp cinnamon
1 cup milk (skim, almond, or soy)
½ banana
1 cup coffee or green tea
1 cup water

SNACK
1 cup nonfat yogurt
½ cup grapes
1 cup water

LUNCH
1 tbsp all natural Smucker's peanut butter on 1 slice whole grain bread
1 tsp honey
1 apple sliced
1 bottle water, diet soda, or green tea

SNACK
1 serving Smart'n Healthy popcorn (1/3 of a bag)
1 cup water

DINNER
4 oz baked or grilled salmon
½ cup whole grain pasta with tomato sauce
1 medium – large salad with 1 or 2 tbsp light salad dressing
1 bottle of water, diet soda, or green tea

DESSERT
3 low-fat Chips Ahoy cookies
1 cup milk (skim, almond, soy)

WEEK 1 DAY 3

BREAKFAST

1 cup Kashi cereal
1 cup milk
½ apple sliced
1 cup coffee or green tea
1 cup water

SNACK

1 Kashi bar
1 cup water

LUNCH

1 slice whole wheat bread
2 slices low-fat cheese
1 medium salad
1 tbsp light salad dressing
1 bottle water

SNACK

½ apple
10 almonds
1 cup water

DINNER

4 oz turkey burger on whole wheat bun
½ plate green beans
Mustard, ketchup, salsa, or light mayonnaise
1 bottle water, diet soda, or green tea

DESSERT

6 oz nonfat yogurt
½ cup fruit
1 cup decaffeinated tea

WEEK 1 DAY 4

BREAKFAST
2 egg whites scrambled
1 slice whole wheat toast
1 fruit serving (Ex. 1/2 grapefruit)
1 cup milk
1 cup coffee or tea
1 cup water

SNACK
6 oz nonfat yogurt
½ cup fruit
1 cup water

LUNCH
Tuna and Tomato Wheel (recipe on page 98).
1 medium to large salad with 1-2 tbsp light salad dressing
1 bottle water

SNACK
½ apple
10 almonds
1 cup water

DINNER
4 oz baked or grilled chicken breast
½ - 1 cup mashed potatoes
½ plate steamed carrots
1 bottle water

DESSERT
1 Eddy's frozen coconut bar
1 cup milk

WEEK 1 DAY 5

BREAKFAST

½ cup oatmeal (made with one cup of water)
Truvia or choice of sweetener and sprinkle with 1 tsp cinnamon
½ banana
1 cup milk
1 cup coffee or tea
1 cup water

SNACK

1 kashi bar
1 cup water

LUNCH

1 bowl chicken noodle soup (deli or restaurant)
1 medium to large mixed salad with 1-2 tbsp light dressing
1 bottle water

SNACK

3 low-fat Chips Ahoy cookies
1 cup water

DINNER

4 oz BBQ chicken breast
1 small corn on the cob
½ plate steamed broccoli (use BBQ sauce for dunking)
1 bottle water (try ¼ lite cranberry juice plus ¾ water)

DESSERT

1 Jala bar
1 cup milk

WEEK 1 DAY 6

BREAKFAST
1 cup cereal
1 cup milk
½ banana
1 cup coffee or tea
1 cup water

SNACK
6 oz nonfat yogurt
½ banana
1 cup water

LUNCH
4 oz grilled chicken breast on whole wheat bun
Ketchup, mustard, or light mayonnaise
10 celery sticks
1 tbsp olive oil and balsamic vinegar
1 bottle water

SNACK
Fruit (1 cup of grapes)
1 cup water

DINNER
1 cup multigrain pasta
½ cup tomato sauce
1 medium to large mixed salad
1 or 2 tbsp light salad dressing
1 bottle water

DESSERT
6 oz nonfat yogurt with fruit
1 cup decaffeinated tea

WEEK 1 DAY 7

BREAKFAST
1 and ½ slice of Cinnamon French Toast (recipe on page 98)
1 oz light maple syrup
1 serving of fruit (Ex. ½ sliced apple)
1 cup milk
1 cup coffee or tea
1 cup water

SNACK
1 Kashi bar
½ apple sliced
1 cup water

LUNCH
2 slices turkey breast on 1 slice whole wheat bread
1 medium to large salad
1 - 2 tbsp light dressing
1 bottle water

SNACK
3 low fat Chips Ahoy cookies
1 cup water

DINNER
4 oz lean beef
½ cup mashed potatoes or ½ baked potato
½ plate boiled green beans
1 bottle water

DESSERT
1 Jala bar
1 cup milk

WEEK 2

GROCERY LIST

Always have the following on hand:

- ☐ Aluminum foil
- ☐ Basil
- ☐ BBQ sauce
- ☐ Bottles of water (16.9 FL OZ - 24 pack).
- ☐ Cinnamon
- ☐ Coffee
- ☐ Extra virgin olive oil
- ☐ Fresh black pepper
- ☐ Garlic powder
- ☐ Green tea
- ☐ Ground flaxseeds (organic)
- ☐ Ketchup
- ☐ Light cranberry juice
- ☐ Light mayonnaise
- ☐ Light salad dressing
- ☐ Mustard
- ☐ Nonstick spray

- ☐ Oregano
- ☐ Organic honey
- ☐ Rice vinegar or Balsamic
- ☐ Small, medium, and large size reusable plastic containers
- ☐ Truvia (or sweetener of choice)
- ☐ Water (1 gallon - purified)

....

- ☐ Eggs (organic brown)
- ☐ Light cheese shredded (Mexican blend)
- ☐ Light cream cheese
- ☐ Light sour cream
- ☐ Milk (skim, soy, almond, or flaxseed)
- ☐ Mozzarella cheese

- ☐ Granola low-fat (Heartland)
- ☐ Whole wheat bagels
- ☐ Whole wheat double fiber bread

- ☐ Apples (organic)
- ☐ Bananas
- ☐ Oranges
- ☐ Strawberries
- ☐ Watermelon chunks

- ☐ 1 green pepper
- ☐ 1 potato or sweet potato

- ☐ 1 red pepper
- ☐ 1 yellow pepper
- ☐ Baby carrots
- ☐ Broccoli
- ☐ Mixed vegetables
- ☐ Mushrooms (white)
- ☐ Sweet onion (1)
- ☐ Romaine lettuce (2 packages)
- ☐ Spinach
- ☐ Tomatoes (4)

- ☐ Chicken noodle soup (deli or restaurant)
- ☐ Lean ground sirloin
- ☐ Mahi Mahi
- ☐ Roast beef (¼ lb sliced)
- ☐ Salmon
- ☐ Turkey breast (¼ lb sliced)

- ☐ Cashews
- ☐ Kashi Chewy Granola Bars
- ☐ Oreo cookies low-fat
- ☐ Pringles potato chips 100 calorie pack
- ☐ Weight Watchers brownies
- ☐ Wheat crackers
- ☐ Wheat tortillas
- ☐ Whole grain pasta

- ☐ 1 jar tomato sauce
- ☐ Hummus
- ☐ Light maple syrup
- ☐ Salsa
- ☐ Smucker's organic peanut butter

WEEK 2 DAY 1

BREAKFAST
1 egg (use nonstick spray if fried)
1 slice whole wheat toast
1 fruit serving (Ex. ½ banana)
1 cup milk
1 cup coffee or tea
1 cup water

SNACK
1 Kashi bar
1 cup water

LUNCH
2 slices roast beef on 1 slice whole wheat bread
Mustard, ketchup, or light mayonnaise
Medium to large mixed vegetable salad
1 tbsp light salad dressing
1 bottle water

SNACK
½ banana
10 cashews
1 cup water (try 1 cup of green tea for energy boost)

DINNER
4 oz baked or grilled salmon
½ cup brown rice
½ plate steamed spinach
1 bottle water (try adding ¼ light cranberry juice to
¾ cup of water)

DESSERT
1 Jala bar
1 cup milk

WEEK 2 DAY 2

BREAKFAST
½ cup low-fat granola (Heartland)
1 cup milk (Skim, Almond, soy, or Flaxseed)
½ apple sliced
1 cup coffee or tea
1 cup water

SNACK
6 oz nonfat yogurt
½ apple sliced
1 cup water

LUNCH
2 slices low-fat cheese
1 slice whole wheat bread
 Add mustard or light mayonnaise
1 orange sliced
1 bottle water

SNACK
1 serving Smart'n Healthy popcorn (1/3 of a bag)
1 cup water

DINNER
4 oz lean ground sirloin grilled on 1 whole wheat bun
Lettuce, tomato, and onion
Mustard, ketchup, or light mayonnaise
½ plate green beans
1 bottle water

DESSERT
1 Jala bar
1 cup milk

WEEK 2 DAY 3

BREAKFAST
>2 egg whites
>1 slice whole wheat toast
>Salsa or ketchup
>1 cup milk
>½ orange
>1 cup coffee or tea
>1 cup water

SNACK
>1 kashi bar
>1 cup water

LUNCH
>2 slices turkey breast on 1 slice whole wheat bread
>Mustard, ketchup, or light mayonnaise
>1 medium to large salad (1 tbsp light salad dressing)
>1 bottle water

SNACK
>5 whole wheat crackers topped with hummus (1 tbsp)
>1 cup water

DINNER
>4 oz Mahi Mahi baked or grilled
>½ baked potato or sweet potato (can add ½ teaspoon
>of Promise spread or light butter)
>½ plate steamed mixed vegetables
>1 bottle water

DESSERT
>6 oz nonfat yogurt
>½ orange sliced

WEEK 2 DAY 4

BREAKFAST

Cinnamon French toast 1 and ½ slice (recipe on page 98)
1 oz light maple syrup
½ banana
1 cup milk (unsweetened almond milk has 30 calories vs. skim milk which has 90 calories)
1 cup coffee or tea
1 cup water

SNACK

½ banana
1 cup water

LUNCH

2 oz chicken salad (recipe on page 99)
1 slice whole wheat bread
Medium to large salad
Add 1 tbsp extra virgin olive oil and balsamic vinegar/rice vinegar
1 bottle water

SNACK

10 cashews
1 cup water

DINNER

4 oz Chicken Parmesan (recipe on page 101)
½ cup pasta whole grain with tomato sauce
½ plate steamed broccoli
1 bottle water

DESSERT

1 Weight Watchers brownie
1 cup milk

WEEK 2 DAY 5

BREAKFAST
 ½ cup low-fat granola (Heartland)
 ½ banana
 1 cup milk
 1 cup coffee or tea
 1 cup water

SNACK
 1 nonfat yogurt 6 oz
 1 cup water

LUNCH
 1 bowl chicken noodle soup (Deli or restaurant)
 1 medium to large salad
 1 tbsp light dressing
 1 bottle water

SNACK
 3 low-fat Oreo cookies
 1 cup water

DINNER
 Chicken Fajitas (recipe on page 99)
 ½ plate steamed white mushrooms
 1 bottle water

DESSERT
 1 Weight Watchers brownie
 1 cup milk

WEEK 2 DAY 6

BREAKFAST

½ whole wheat bagel
1 tbsp light cream cheese
1 cup milk
½ banana
1 cup coffee or tea
1 cup water

SNACK

1 cup nonfat yogurt
1 cup water

LUNCH

½ whole wheat bagel
1 tbsp light cream cheese
1 medium to large salad
1 tbsp extra virgin olive oil
1 tbsp vinegar
1 bottle water

SNACK

100 calorie pack Pringles potato chips
1 cup water

DINNER

4 oz salmon (baked or grilled)
½ cup whole grain pasta (add tomato sauce)
½ plate tomato, onion, and cucumber salad (recipe on page 99)
1 bottle water

DESSERT

1 Jala bar
1 cup milk

WEEK 2 DAY 7

BREAKFAST
½ whole wheat bagel
1 tsp organic honey
1 tbsp organic all natural Smucker's peanut butter
½ cup strawberries
1 cup milk
1 cup coffee or tea

SNACK
1 Kashi bar (Chewy Granola)
1 cup water

LUNCH
2 slices of roast beef
1 slice whole wheat bread
1 medium to large salad (1 tbsp light dressing)
1 bottle water

SNACK
100 calorie pack Pringles potato chips
1 cup water

DINNER
4 oz grilled chicken on a whole wheat bun
Lettuce, tomato, and onion
Mustard, ketchup, or light mayonnaise
½ plate steamed mixed vegetables
1 bottle water

DESSERT
3 low-fat Oreo cookies
1 cup milk

WEEK 3

GROCERY LIST

Always have the following on hand:

- ☐ Bottles of water (16.9 FL OZ - 24 pack).
- ☐ Water (1 gallon - purified)
- ☐ Coffee
- ☐ Green tea
- ☐ Light salad dressing
- ☐ Rice vinegar or Balsamic
- ☐ Nonstick spray
- ☐ Extra virgin olive oil
- ☐ Light cranberry juice
- ☐ Ground flaxseeds (organic)
- ☐ Cinnamon
- ☐ Fresh black pepper
- ☐ Garlic powder
- ☐ Basil
- ☐ Oregano
- ☐ Mustard
- ☐ BBQ sauce

☐ Ketchup
☐ Light mayonnaise
☐ Organic honey
☐ Truvia (or sweetener of choice)
☐ Aluminum foil
☐ Small, medium, and large size reusable plastic containers
☐ Eggs (organic brown)
☐ Milk (skim, soy, almond, or flaxseed)
☐ Mozzarella cheese
☐ Yogurt (1 nonfat 6 oz)

☐ Brown rice
☐ Cream of Wheat
☐ Kashi cereal Go Lean Crunch
☐ Wheat English muffins
☐ Whole grain pasta
☐ Whole wheat double fiber bread

☐ Apples (organic)
☐ Bananas
☐ Watermelon chunks

☐ 1 green pepper
☐ 1 red pepper
☐ 1 yellow pepper
☐ Baby carrots
☐ Broccoli
☐ Celery sticks

- ☐ Green beans
- ☐ Mixed vegetables
- ☐ Sweet onion (1)
- ☐ Romaine lettuce (2 packages)
- ☐ Tomatoes (4)
- ☐ Albacore tuna (1 can)
- ☐ Chicken breast
- ☐ Ground beef (lean)
- ☐ Roast beef (¼ pound)
- ☐ Salmon
- ☐ Tilapia
- ☐ Turkey breast (¼ lb sliced)
- ☐ Turkey burgers (extra lean)

- ☐ Jala bars (frozen low-fat yogurt)
- ☐ Low-fat Oreo cookies
- ☐ Pretzels
- ☐ Roasted almonds (no salt)
- ☐ Smart'n Healthy popcorn

- ☐ 1 jar tomato sauce
- ☐ Hummus
- ☐ Salsa
- ☐ Seasoned bread crumbs
- ☐ Smucker's organic peanut butter
- ☐ Tortillas (wheat)

WEEK 3 DAY 1

BREAKFAST

½ cup dry oat meal cooked in 1 cup water
Add 1 tsp ground flaxseeds
½ banana
1 cup milk
1 cup coffee or tea
1 cup water

SNACK

10 almonds
1 cup water

LUNCH

1 slice whole wheat bread
1 tbsp peanut butter
1 tsp organic honey
1 apple sliced
1 bottle water

SNACK

10 celery sticks with 1 tbsp light salad dressing
1 cup water

DINNER

Fried chicken with seasoned bread crumbs (recipe on page 100)
½ cup brown rice
½ plate steamed broccoli
1 bottle water

DESSERT

1 Jala bar
1 cup milk

WEEK 3 DAY 2

BREAKFAST

1 cup Cream of Wheat (add 1 tsp ground flaxseeds)

½ banana

1 cup milk

1 cup coffee or tea

1 cup water

SNACK

10 almonds

1 cup water

LUNCH

Left over fried chicken with seasoned bread crumbs
(2 - 4 oz)

½ cup brown rice

Steamed mixed vegetables

1 bottle water

SNACK

Smart'n Healthy popcorn (1/3 of a bag)

1 cup water

DINNER

Turkey burger on whole wheat bun

1 medium to large salad

1 tbsp light salad dressing

1 bottle water

DESSERT

3 low-fat Oreo cookies

1 cup milk

WEEK 3 DAY 3

BREAKFAST
2 egg whites scrambled with salsa
1 slice whole wheat bread
1 tsp light cream cheese
½ apple
1 cup milk
1 cup coffee or tea
1 cup water

SNACK
10 almonds
1 cup water

LUNCH
½ tuna sandwich with lettuce, tomato, and onion on whole wheat bread
1 medium to large salad
1 tbsp extra virgin olive oil and vinegar
1 bottle water

SNACK
1 serving of pretzels
1 cup water
1 cup green tea for energy boost

DINNER
Chicken fajitas (recipe on page 99)
Sautee spinach with mushrooms in small amount of extra virgin olive oil
1 bottle water (option: ¼ light cranberry juice and ¾ water)

DESSERT
1 Jala bar
1 cup milk

WEEK 3 DAY 4

BREAKFAST
1 cup Kashi cereal Go Lean Crunch
1 cup milk
½ banana
1 cup coffee or tea
1 cup water

SNACK
10 almonds
1 cup water

LUNCH
1 slice whole wheat bread
2 slices turkey breast
Mustard, ketchup, or light mayonnaise
20 baby carrots with 1 tbsp light salad dressing
1 bottle water

SNACK
10 celery sticks with 1 tbsp hummus
1 cup water

DINNER
4 oz tilapia baked
½ cup pasta with tomato sauce
½ plate green beans
1 bottle water

DESSERT
1 Jala bar
1 cup milk

WEEK 3 DAY 5

BREAKFAST

Good Morning Sandwich (recipe on page 97)
½ cup watermelon chunks (6 pieces)
1 cup milk
1 cup coffee or tea
1 cup water

SNACK

10 almonds
1 cup water

LUNCH

2 slices roast beef
1 slice whole wheat bread
Mustard, ketchup, or light mayonnaise
10 celery sticks with 1 tbsp hummus
1 bottle water

SNACK

1 serving of pretzels
1 cup water
1 cup green tea for energy boost (can add zero calorie sweeteners)

DINNER

1 cup spaghetti with tomato sauce
Two 2 oz meatballs
½ plate steamed broccoli
1 bottle water

DESSERT

3 low-fat Oreo cookies
1 cup milk

WEEK 3 DAY 6

BREAKFAST
2 egg whites scrambled
1 slice whole wheat toast with ½ tsp light butter
½ banana
1 cup milk
1 cup coffee or tea
1 cup water

SNACK
10 almonds
1 cup water

LUNCH
1 slice whole wheat bread with 1 tbsp peanut butter
and 1 tsp honey
1 apple sliced
1 bottle water (option: ¼ light cranberry juice and ¾
bottle water)

SNACK
Smart'n Healthy popcorn (1/3 of a bag)
1 cup water
1 cup green tea

DINNER
4 oz baked salmon
½ cup brown rice
½ plate steamed mixed vegetables
1 bottle water

DESSERT
3 low-fat Oreo cookies
1 cup milk
1 cup decaffeinated coffee

WEEK 3 DAY 7

BREAKFAST

Cinnamon French toast 1 and ½ slices (recipe on page 98)
1 oz light maple syrup
½ apple
1 cup milk
1 cup coffee or tea

SNACK

1 nonfat yogurt 6 oz
1 cup water

LUNCH

4 oz baked salmon
½ cup brown rice
½ plate steamed mixed vegetables
1 bottle water

SNACK

3 low-fat Oreo cookies
1 cup green tea for energy boost
1 cup water

DINNER

4 oz chicken parmesan (recipe on page 101)
1 medium to large salad with 1 tbsp extra virgin olive oil and vinegar
1 cup water

DESSERT

1 Jala bar
1 cup milk

WEEK 4

GROCERY LIST

Always have the following on hand:

- ☐ Bottles of water (16.9 FL OZ - 24 pack).
- ☐ Water (1 gallon - purified)
- ☐ Coffee
- ☐ Green tea
- ☐ Light salad dressing
- ☐ Rice vinegar or Balsamic
- ☐ Nonstick spray
- ☐ Extra virgin olive oil
- ☐ Light cranberry juice
- ☐ Ground flaxseeds (organic)
- ☐ Cinnamon
- ☐ Fresh black pepper
- ☐ Garlic powder
- ☐ Basil
- ☐ Oregano
- ☐ Mustard
- ☐ BBQ sauce
- ☐ Ketchup

- ☐ Light mayonnaise
- ☐ Organic honey
- ☐ Truvia (or sweetener of choice)
- ☐ Aluminum foil
- ☐ Small, medium, and large size reusable plastic containers

....

- ☐ Eggs (organic brown)
- ☐ Milk (skim, soy, almond, or flaxseed)
- ☐ Orange juice
- ☐ Yogurt (1 nonfat 6 oz)

- ☐ Kashi cereal Go Lean Crunch
- ☐ Oatmeal bread
- ☐ Whole grain pasta
- ☐ Whole wheat buns

- ☐ Apples (organic)
- ☐ Bananas
- ☐ Cherries
- ☐ Grapes

- ☐ 1 baked potato/sweet potato
- ☐ 1 green pepper
- ☐ 1 red pepper
- ☐ 1 yellow pepper
- ☐ 2 cucumbers

- ☐ Asparagus
- ☐ Baby carrots
- ☐ Celery sticks
- ☐ Green beans
- ☐ Sweet onion (1)
- ☐ Romaine lettuce (2 packages)
- ☐ Tomatoes (4)
- ☐ Vegetable soup (Deli or restaurant)

- ☐ Albacore tuna (1 can)
- ☐ Chicken breast
- ☐ Roast beef (¼ pound)
- ☐ Salmon
- ☐ Tilapia
- ☐ Turkey breast (¼ lb sliced)
- ☐ Turkey burgers (extra lean)

- ☐ 1 jar tomato sauce
- ☐ Cashews
- ☐ Eddy's frozen coconut bars (or other fruit bar to liking)
- ☐ Hummus
- ☐ Jala bars (frozen low-fat yogurt)
- ☐ Low-fat Chips Ahoy cookies
- ☐ Tortillas (wheat)
- ☐ Doritos 100 calorie pack

WEEK 4 DAY 1

BREAKFAST

Oatmeal (add 1 tsp ground flaxseed)
½ cup grapes
1 cup milk
1 cup coffee or tea
1 cup water

SNACK

10 cashews
1 cup water

LUNCH

2 slices turkey breast on 1 slice oatmeal bread
Mustard, ketchup, or light mayonnaise
1 medium to large salad with 1 tbsp oil and vinegar
salad dressing
1 bottle water

SNACK

3 low-fat Chips Ahoy cookies
1 cup water
1 cup green tea for energy boost (no sugar)

DINNER

4 oz baked chicken breast
½ cup whole wheat pasta with tomato sauce
½ plate steamed broccoli
1 bottle water

DESSERT

1 Eddy's frozen coconut bar
1 cup milk

WEEK 4 DAY 2

BREAKFAST

1 cup Cream of Wheat (add 1 tsp ground flaxseeds)

½ cup grapes

1 cup milk

1 cup coffee or tea

1 cup water

SNACK

10 cashews

1 cup water

LUNCH

2 to 4 oz leftover chicken

½ cup whole wheat pasta

1 medium to large salad with 1 tbsp low-fat dressing

1 bottle water

SNACK

Doritos 100 calorie pack

1 cup water

DINNER

4 oz chicken breast on whole wheat bun

Lettuce, tomato, and onion

Mustard, ketchup, or light mayonnaise

1 medium to large salad with 1 tbsp low-fat salad dressing

1 bottle water

DESSERT

3 low-fat Chips Ahoy cookies

1 cup milk

WEEK 4 DAY 3

BREAKFAST
2 egg whites scrambled top with salsa
1 slice oatmeal bread with 1 tsp light cream cheese
½ cup cherries
1 cup milk
1 cup coffee or tea
1 cup water

SNACK
10 cashews
1 cup water

LUNCH
2 slices roast beef on 1 slice oatmeal bread
Mustard, ketchup, or light mayonnaise
20 baby carrots with 1 tbsp light salad dressing
1 bottle water

SNACK
Doritos 100 calorie pack
1 cup water
1 cup green tea for energy boost

DINNER
4 oz tilapia with seasoned bread crumbs baked or fried (recipe on page 100)
½ baked potato/sweet potato
½ teaspoon light butter and ½ teaspoon light sour cream
½ plate green beans
1 bottle water (option: 1/4 light cranberry juice and ¾ water)

DESSERT
3 low-fat Chips Ahoy
1 cup milk

WEEK 4 DAY 4

BREAKFAST
1 cup Kashi cereal Go Lean Crunch
1 cup milk
½ cup cherries
1 cup coffee or tea
1 cup water

SNACK
10 cashews
1 cup water

LUNCH
4 oz left over tilapia
½ baked potato/sweet potato
½ teaspoon light butter
½ teaspoon light sour cream
1 medium to large salad with 1 tbsp light salad dressing
1 bottle water

SNACK
10 celery sticks with 1 tbsp hummus
1 cup water

DINNER
Chicken fajitas (recipe on page 99)
½ plate steamed spinach
1 bottle water

DESSERT
1 Jala bar
1 cup milk
1 cup decaffeinated tea

WEEK 4 DAY 5

BREAKFAST
1 cup oatmeal (add 1 tsp ground flaxseeds)
4 oz orange juice
1 cup milk
1 cup coffee or tea
1 cup water

SNACK
½ apple
10 cashews
1 cup water

LUNCH
Egg salad (recipe on page 101)
1 slice oatmeal bread
½ plate green beans
1 bottle water

SNACK
½ apple
10 cashews
1 cup water

DINNER
1 cup whole wheat pasta with tomato sauce
½ plate steamed asparagus
1 bottle water

DESSERT
1 Jala bar
1 cup milk

WEEK 4 DAY 6

BREAKFAST
>1 cup Kashi cereal Go Lean Crunch
>½ banana
>1 cup milk
>1 cup coffee or tea
>1 cup water

SNACK
>½ banana
>10 cashews
>1 cup water

LUNCH
>1 tbsp peanut butter
>1 slice oatmeal bread
>1 tsp organic honey
>1 apple sliced
>1 bottle water (option: 1/4 light cranberry juice and ¾ water)

SNACK
>Smart'n Healthy popcorn (1/3 of bag)
>1 cup water

DINNER
>4 oz turkey burger on whole wheat bun with lettuce, tomato, and onion
>Mustard, ketchup, or light mayonnaise
>½ plate green beans
>1 bottle water

DESSERT
>6 oz yogurt
>½ cup mixed fruit

WEEK 4 DAY 7

BREAKFAST

Good Morning Sandwich (recipe on page 97)
½ banana
1 cup milk
1 cup coffee or tea
1 cup water

SNACK

1 Kashi bar (Chewy Granola)
1 cup water

LUNCH

2 oz tuna salad
1 slice oatmeal bread
1 medium to large salad with 1 tbsp low-fat salad dressing
1 bottle water

SNACK

½ banana
1 cup water
1 cup decaffeinated coffee

DINNER

4 oz broiled salmon
½ cup brown rice
1 bowl of vegetable soup (Deli or restaurant)
1 bottle water

DESSERT

1 Eddy's frozen coconut bar
1 cup milk

WEEK 5

GROCERY LIST

Always have the following on hand:

- ☐ Bottles of water (16.9 FL OZ - 24 pack).
- ☐ Water (1 gallon - purified)
- ☐ Coffee
- ☐ Green tea
- ☐ Light salad dressing
- ☐ Rice vinegar or Balsamic
- ☐ Nonstick spray
- ☐ Extra virgin olive oil
- ☐ Light cranberry juice
- ☐ Ground flaxseeds (organic)
- ☐ Cinnamon
- ☐ Fresh black pepper
- ☐ Garlic powder
- ☐ Basil
- ☐ Oregano
- ☐ Mustard
- ☐ BBQ sauce

- ☐ Ketchup
- ☐ Light mayonnaise
- ☐ Organic honey
- ☐ Truvia (or sweetener of choice)
- ☐ Aluminum foil
- ☐ Small, medium, and large size reusable plastic containers

---

- ☐ Milk (skim, soy, almond, or flaxseed)
- ☐ Mozzarella cheese
- ☐ Yogurt (4 nonfat 6 oz)

- ☐ Cream of Wheat
- ☐ English muffins whole wheat
- ☐ Kashi cereal Go Lean Crunch
- ☐ Oatmeal bread

- ☐ Apples (organic)
- ☐ Bananas
- ☐ Grapes
- ☐ Strawberries
- ☐ 1 baked potato/sweet potato
- ☐ Asparagus
- ☐ Baby carrots
- ☐ Broccoli
- ☐ Celery sticks
- ☐ Corn on the cob
- ☐ Mushrooms (white)

- ☐ Sweet onion (1)
- ☐ Romaine lettuce (2 packages)
- ☐ Spinach
- ☐ Tomatoes (4)
- ☐ Vegetable soup (fresh from deli or restaurant)

- ☐ Albacore tuna (1 can)
- ☐ Baked beans (fresh from favorite BBQ restaurant)
- ☐ Chicken breast
- ☐ Lean meat sirloin
- ☐ Roast beef (¼ pound)
- ☐ Salmon
- ☐ Tilapia
- ☐ Tuna steak
- ☐ Turkey breast (¼ lb sliced)
- ☐ Turkey burgers (extra lean)

- ☐ Eddy's frozen coconut bars (or other fruit bar to liking)
- ☐ Jala bars (frozen low-fat yogurt)
- ☐ Kashi bars (Chewy Granola)
- ☐ Pretzels 100 calorie pack
- ☐ Smart'n Healthy popcorn
- ☐ 1 jar tomato sauce
- ☐ 1 cheese pizza (buy fresh on the day to be eaten. Leftovers can be frozen for later use)
- ☐ Kosher dill pickles
- ☐ Pistachios (no salt)

WEEK 5 DAY 1

BREAKFAST
Cinnamon French toast (recipe on page 98)
1 oz light maple syrup
½ cup strawberries
1 cup milk
1 cup coffee or tea
1 cup water

SNACK
½ cup strawberries
10 pistachios
1 cup water

LUNCH
1 slice oatmeal bread
2 slices turkey breast
Mustard, ketchup, or light mayonnaise
10 celery sticks with 1 tbsp low-fat salad dressing
1 bottle water

SNACK
Smart'n Healthy popcorn (1/3 of a bag)
1 cup water

DINNER
4 oz baked chicken breast
½ cup whole wheat pasta with tomato sauce
½ plate steamed spinach and mushrooms
1 bottle water

DESSERT
6 oz nonfat yogurt
½ cup fruit

WEEK 5 DAY 2

BREAKFAST
1 cup oatmeal (add 1 tsp ground flaxseeds)
½ cup strawberries
1 cup milk
1 cup coffee or tea
1 cup water

SNACK
1 Kashi bar (Chewy Granola)
1 cup water

LUNCH
2 slices roast beef on 1 slice oatmeal bread
Mustard, ketchup, or light mayonnaise
1 kosher dill pickle
1 bottle water

SNACK
Pretzels 100 calorie pack
1 cup water

DINNER
4 oz baked salmon
½ cup brown rice
½ plate steamed carrots
1 bottle water

DESSERT
1 Jala bar
1 cup milk

WEEK 5 DAY 3

BREAKFAST

Good Morning Sandwich (recipe on page 97)
½ cup grapes
1 cup milk
1 cup coffee or tea
1 cup water

SNACK

1 Kashi bar (Chewy Granola)
1 cup water

LUNCH

2 tbsp tuna salad on 1 slice oatmeal bread (recipe on page 98)
1 medium to large salad with 1 tbsp light salad dressing
1 bottle water

SNACK

Pretzels 100 calorie pack
1 cup water

DINNER

4 oz sliced sirloin
½ baked potato or sweet potato
½ tsp light butter and ½ tsp light sour cream
½ plate steamed asparagus
1 bottle water

DESSERT

1 Jala bar
1 cup milk

WEEK 5 DAY 4

BREAKFAST
1 cup Kashi cereal Go Lean Crunch
½ banana
1 cup milk
1 cup coffee or tea
1 cup water

SNACK
½ banana
10 pistachios
1 cup water

LUNCH
1 slice oatmeal bread
1 tbsp peanut butter
1 tsp honey
1 apple sliced
1 bottle water

SNACK
10 celery sticks with 1 tbsp low-fat dressing
1 cup water

DINNER
Turkey burger on English muffin
Lettuce, tomato, and onion
1 medium to large salad with 1 tbsp extra virgin olive
oil and vinegar
1 bottle water

DESSERT
1 Eddy's frozen coconut bar
1 cup milk

WEEK 5 DAY 5

BREAKFAST

   2 egg whites scrambled
   1 slice oatmeal bread toast
   ½ banana
   1 cup milk
   1 cup coffee or tea
   1 cup water

SNACK

   ½ banana
   10 pistachios
   1 cup water

LUNCH

   1 cup whole wheat pasta with ½ cup tomato sauce
   1 medium to large salad with 1 tbsp light salad dressing
   1 bottle water

SNACK

   Smart'n Balance popcorn (1/3 of a bag)
   1 cup water

DINNER

   4 oz tilapia
   ½ cup brown rice
   ½ plate steamed broccoli
   1 bottle water

DESSERT

   6 oz nonfat yogurt
   ½ cup fruit

WEEK 5 DAY 6

BREAKFAST
1 cup Kashi cereal Go Lean Crunch
½ apple
1 cup milk
1 cup coffee or tea
1 cup water

SNACK
1 kashi bar (Chewy Granola)
1 cup water

LUNCH
1 slice cheese pizza
1 medium to large salad with 1 tbsp extra virgin olive oil and vinegar
1 bottle water

SNACK
½ cup frozen yogurt
½ cup strawberries
1 cup water

DINNER
4 oz BBQ chicken breast
1 small corn on the cob
½ cup baked beans
1 medium to large salad with 1 tbsp low-fat salad dressing
1 bottle water

DESSERT
1 Jala bar
1 cup milk

WEEK 5 DAY 7

BREAKFAST
1 bowl Cream of Wheat (add 1 tsp ground flaxseeds)
½ apple
1 cup milk
1 cup coffee or tea
1 cup water

SNACK
1 Kashi bar (Chewy Granola)
1 cup water

LUNCH
4 oz grilled tuna or chicken breast
1 whole wheat bun or 1 slice of oatmeal bread
Lettuce, tomato, and onion
Mustard, ketchup, or light mayonnaise
1 medium to large salad with 1 tbsp extra virgin olive
oil and vinegar dressing
1 bottle water

SNACK
6 oz nonfat yogurt
1 cup water

DINNER
4 oz chicken parmesan
½ cup whole wheat pasta with tomato sauce
1 bowl fresh vegetable soup
1 bottle water

DESSERT
1 Eddy's frozen coconut/ fruit bar
1 cup milk

WEEK 6

GROCERY LIST

Always have the following on hand:

- [ ] Bottles of water (16.9 FL OZ - 24 pack)
- [ ] Water (1 gallon - purified)
- [ ] Coffee
- [ ] Green tea
- [ ] Light salad dressing
- [ ] Rice vinegar or Balsamic
- [ ] Nonstick spray
- [ ] Extra virgin olive oil
- [ ] Light cranberry juice
- [ ] Ground flaxseeds (organic)
- [ ] Cinnamon
- [ ] Fresh black pepper
- [ ] Garlic powder
- [ ] Basil
- [ ] Oregano
- [ ] Mustard
- [ ] BBQ sauce
- [ ] Ketchup

- ☐ Light mayonnaise
- ☐ Organic honey
- ☐ Truvia (or sweetener of choice)
- ☐ Aluminum foil
- ☐ Small, medium, and large size reusable plastic containers

....

- ☐ Eggs (organic)
- ☐ Milk (skim, soy, almond, or flaxseed)
- ☐ Mozzarella cheese
- ☐ Nonfat whip cream
- ☐ Yogurt (1 nonfat 6 oz)

- ☐ Kashi cereal Go Lean Crunch
- ☐ Multi grain pasta
- ☐ Oatmeal bread

- ☐ Apples (organic)
- ☐ Bananas
- ☐ Watermelon chunks

- ☐ 1 baked potato/sweet potato
- ☐ Asparagus
- ☐ Baby carrots
- ☐ Broccoli
- ☐ Cucumbers (2)
- ☐ Green beans

- ☐ Mushrooms portabella
- ☐ Sweet onion (1)
- ☐ Romaine lettuce (2 packages)
- ☐ Spinach
- ☐ Tomatoes (4)
- ☐ Vegetable soup (fresh from deli or restaurant)

- ☐ Albacore tuna (2 cans)
- ☐ Chicken breast
- ☐ Lean meat sirloin
- ☐ Roast beef (¼ pound)
- ☐ Salmon
- ☐ Tilapia
- ☐ Turkey breast (¼ lb sliced)

- ☐ Jala bars (frozen low-fat yogurt)
- ☐ Cashews (no salt)
- ☐ Pretzels 100 calorie pack
- ☐ Pringles potato chips 100 calorie pack
- ☐ 1 jar tomato sauce

WEEK 6 DAY 1

BREAKFAST

Good Morning Sandwich (recipe on page 97)
½ cup watermelon
1 cup milk
1 cup coffee or tea
1 cup water

SNACK

½ cup watermelon
10 cashews
1 cup water

LUNCH

3 slices turkey breast on 1 slice oatmeal bread
Mustard, ketchup, or light mayonnaise
20 baby carrots with light salad dressing
1 bottle water

SNACK

Pringles potato chips 100 calorie pack
1 cup water

DINNER

4 oz baked or grilled salmon
½ cup whole grain pasta with tomato sauce
½ plate steamed spinach with mushrooms
1 bottle water

DESSERT

6 oz nonfat yogurt
½ cup of fruit

WEEK 6 DAY 2

BREAKFAST

1 cup oatmeal (add 1 teaspoon of ground flaxseeds)
½ cup watermelon
1 cup milk
1 cup coffee or tea
1 cup water

SNACK

½ cup watermelon
10 cashews
1 cup water

LUNCH

3 slices of roast beef on 1 slice oatmeal bread
Mustard, ketchup, or light mayonnaise
1 kosher dill pickle
1 bottle water

SNACK

Pringles potato chips 100 calorie pack
1 cup water

DINNER

4 oz baked chicken breast with BBQ sauce
½ baked potato or ½ sweet potato
½ plate steamed broccoli
1 bottle water

DESERT

1 Jala bar
1 cup milk

WEEK 6 DAY 3

BREAKFAST
1 serving of Cream of Wheat (add 1 tsp ground flaxseeds)
½ apple
1 cup milk
1 cup coffee or tea
1 cup water

SNACK
½ apple
10 cashews
1 cup water

LUNCH
2 tbsp tuna salad
1 slice oatmeal bread
1 medium to large salad with 1 tbsp extra virgin olive oil and vinegar salad dressing
1 bottle water

SNACK
Pretzels 100 calorie pack
1 cup water

DINNER
4 oz sliced sirloin
½ baked potato or ½ sweet potato
½ plate steamed asparagus
1 bottle water

DESSERT
1 Jala bar
1 cup milk

WEEK 6 DAY 4

BREAKFAST
2 egg whites scrambled
1 slice oatmeal bread
½ apple
1 cup milk
1 cup coffee/tea
1 cup water

SNACK
½ apple
10 cashews
1 cup water

LUNCH
3 slices turkey breast on 1 slice oatmeal bread
Mustard, ketchup, or light mayonnaise
1 large kosher dill pickle
1 bottle water

SNACK
Pringles potato chips 100 calorie pack
1 cup water

DINNER
Fried chicken with Seasoned Bread crumbs (recipe on page 100)
½ cup whole grain pasta with tomato sauce
1 medium to large salad with 1 tbsp light dressing
1 bottle water

DESSERT
200 calorie milkshake (recipe on page 103)

WEEK 6 DAY 5

BREAKFAST

1 cup Kashi cereal

1 cup milk

½ banana

1 cup coffee or tea

1 cup water

SNACK

½ banana

10 cashews

1 cup water

LUNCH

1 cup whole wheat pasta with tomato sauce

½ plate boiled green beans

1 bottle water

SNACK

Pringles potato chips 100 calorie pack

1 cup water

DINNER

4 oz baked tilapia

½ cup brown rice

1 medium to large salad with 1 tbsp vinegar salad dressing

1 bottle water

DESSERT

1 Jala bar

1 cup milk

WEEK 6 DAY 6

BREAKFAST
1 serving oatmeal
½ banana
1 cup milk
1 cup coffee or tea
1 cup water

SNACK
½ banana
10 cashews
1 cup water

LUNCH
1 tuna and tomato wheel (recipe on page 98)
1 tomato, onion, and cucumber salad (recipe on page 99)
1 bottle water

SNACK
Pretzels 100 calorie pack
1 cup water

DINNER
1 slice cheese pizza
½ plate steamed spinach
1 bottle water

DESSERT
1 Jala bar
1 cup milk

WEEK 6 DAY 7

BREAKFAST
2 egg whites scrambled
1 slice of oatmeal bread
½ banana
1 cup milk
1 cup coffee or tea
1 cup water

SNACK
½ banana
10 cashews
1 cup water

LUNCH
1 slice cheese pizza
1 medium to large salad with 1 tbsp extra virgin olive oil and vinegar
1 bottle water

SNACK
1 apple sliced
1 cup water

DINNER
4 oz chicken parmesan (recipe on page 101)
½ cup whole grain pasta with tomato sauce
1 bowl fresh vegetable soup
1 bottle water

DESSERT
6 oz yogurt with ½ cup fruit
2 tbsp nonfat whip cream

WEEK 7

GROCERY LIST

Always have the following on hand:

- [ ] Bottles of water (16.9 FL OZ - 24 pack)
- [ ] Water (1 gallon - purified)
- [ ] Coffee
- [ ] Green tea
- [ ] Light salad dressing
- [ ] Rice vinegar or Balsamic
- [ ] Nonstick spray
- [ ] Extra virgin olive oil
- [ ] Light cranberry juice
- [ ] Ground flaxseeds (organic)
- [ ] Cinnamon
- [ ] Fresh black pepper
- [ ] Garlic powder
- [ ] Basil
- [ ] Oregano
- [ ] Mustard
- [ ] BBQ sauce
- [ ] Ketchup

☐ Light mayonnaise

☐ Organic honey

☐ Truvia (or sweetener of choice)

☐ Aluminum foil

☐ Small, medium, and large size reusable plastic containers

☐ Eggs (organic)

☐ Milk (skim, soy, almond, or flaxseed)

☐ Swiss or cheddar cheese low-fat sliced

☐ Yogurt (1 nonfat 6 oz)

☐ Brown rice

☐ Low-fat granola (Heartland)

☐ Wheat tortilla

☐ Wheatena toasted wheat cereal

☐ Whole grain pasta

☐ Whole wheat bread (double Fiber)

☐ Whole wheat buns

☐ Apples (organic)

☐ Bananas

☐ Grapes

☐ 1 green pepper

☐ 1 red pepper

☐ 2 baked potato/sweet potato

☐ Asparagus

☐ Broccoli
☐ Carrots
☐ Celery sticks
☐ Cucumbers (1)
☐ Green beans
☐ Onion chopped (2 containers)
☐ Romaine lettuce (2 packages)
☐ Tomatoes (5)

☐ Albacore tuna (1 can)
☐ Chicken breast
☐ Salmon
☐ Tilapia
☐ Turkey breast (½ lb sliced)
☐ Turkey burgers extra lean

☐ 1 jar tomato sauce
☐ Baked cheddar goldfish crackers
☐ Kashi Bars (Chewy Granola)
☐ Kashi Chocolate Soft – Baked Squares
☐ Oatmeal cookies (Back to Nature)
☐ Raw almonds no salt
☐ Weight Watchers Ice Cream Bars

☐ Guacamole
☐ Salsa
☐ Seasoned bread crumbs

WEEK 7 DAY 1

BREAKFAST

Wheatena toasted wheat cereal (1 serving) add one tsp ground flaxseeds and sweetener

½ banana

1 cup milk

1 cup coffee or tea

1 cup water

SNACK

1 Kashi bar Chewy Granola

1 cup water

LUNCH

1 tuna and tomato wheel (recipe on page 98)

1 tomato, onion, and cucumber salad (recipe on page 99)

1 bottle water

SNACK

½ banana

5 raw almonds

1 cup water

DINNER

Chicken Fajitas (recipe on page 99)

Steamed broccoli

1 bottle water

DESSERT

1 Kashi Chocolate Soft-Baked Square

1 cup milk

WEEK 7 DAY 2

BREAKFAST

½ cup low-fat granola Heartland

1 cup milk

½ apple

1 cup coffee or tea

1 cup water

SNACK

½ apple

5 raw almonds

1 cup water

LUNCH

½ chicken salad sandwich (recipe on page 99)

1 medium-large salad with 1 tbsp light salad dressing

1 bottle water

SNACK

1 Kashi bar Chewy Granola

1 cup water

DINNER

Fried chicken with seasoned bread crumbs (recipe on page 100)

½ cup brown rice

Steamed carrots

1 bottle water

DESSERT

200 calorie milkshake (recipe on page 103)

WEEK 7 DAY 3

BREAKFAST
1 minute egg sandwich (recipe on page 97)
½ cup grapes
1 cup milk
1 cup coffee or tea
1 cup water

SNACK
1 Kashi bar Chewy Granola
1 cup water

LUNCH
½ egg salad sandwich (recipe on page 101)
1 medium-large salad with 1 tbsp extra virgin olive oil and rice vinegar
1 bottle water

SNACK
½ cup grapes
5 raw almonds
1 cup water

DINNER
Fried tilapia with seasoned bread crumbs (recipe on page 100)
½ baked or sweet potato
½ plate boiled green beans
1 bottle water

DESSERT
1 Weight Watchers Ice cream bar
1 cup milk

WEEK 7 DAY 4

BREAKFAST

Cinnamon French toast (recipe on page 98)
½ banana
1 cup coffee or tea
1 cup water

SNACK

½ banana
5 raw almonds
1 cup water

LUNCH

1 slice whole wheat double fiber
1 tbsp organic peanut butter and 1 tsp organic honey
1 apple
1 bottle water

SNACK

2 oatmeal cookies (Back to Nature)
1 cup water

DINNER

4 oz baked salmon
½ baked or sweet potato
½ plate steamed asparagus
1 bottle water

DESSERT

1 Weight Watchers ice cream bar
1 cup milk

WEEK 7 DAY 5

BREAKFAST
Wheatena toasted cereal (1 serving)
Add 1 tsp ground flaxseed and sweetener
½ apple
1 cup milk

SNACK
1 Kashi bar Chewy Granola
1 cup water

LUNCH
2 slices of turkey breast on 1 slice whole wheat double fiber bread
Mustard, ketchup, or light mayonnaise
1 cup raw carrots
1 bottle water

SNACK
½ apple
5 raw almonds
1 cup water

DINNER
Chicken parmesan (recipe on page 101)
½ cup whole grain pasta with ½ cup tomato sauce
1 medium-large salad with 1 tbsp extra virgin olive oil and rice vinegar
1 bottle water

DESERT
1 Kashi Chocolate Soft-Baked Square
1 cup milk

WEEK 7 DAY 6

BREAKFAST

2 egg whites scrambled
1 slice whole wheat double fiber toast
½ cup grapes
1 cup milk
1 cup coffee or tea
1 cup water

SNACK

6 oz nonfat yogurt
1 cup water

LUNCH

2 slices of low-fat cheese on 1 slice whole wheat double fiber bread
Mustard, ketchup, or light mayonnaise
1 apple
1 bottle water

SNACK

1 package baked cheddar goldfish crackers
1 cup water

DINNER

Turkey burger on whole wheat bun
Lettuce, tomato, and onion
Boiled green beans
1 bottle water

DESSERT

2 oatmeal cookies
1 cup milk

WEEK 7 DAY 7

BREAKFAST
½ cup of low fat granola Heartland
1 cup milk
½ banana
1 cup coffee or tea
1 cup water

SNACK
½ banana
5 raw almonds
1 cup water

LUNCH
½ turkey sandwich
3 slices of turkey
1 slice of whole wheat double fiber bread
1 medium-large salad with 1 tablespoon of light salad dressing
Mustard, ketchup and light mayonnaise
1 bottle water

SNACK
1 package baked cheddar goldfish crackers
1 cup water

DINNER
Eat out at restaurant eat ½ of meal and add side of steamed vegetables
1 glass of water with lemon

DESSERT
Share a dessert with friend or family and 1 cup of decaffeinated coffee

WEEK 8

GROCERY LIST

Always have the following on hand:

☐ Bottles of water (16.9 FL OZ - 24 pack)

☐ Water (1 gallon - purified)

☐ Coffee

☐ Green tea

☐ Light salad dressing

☐ Rice vinegar or Balsamic

☐ Nonstick spray

☐ Extra virgin olive oil

☐ Light cranberry juice

☐ Ground flaxseeds (organic)

☐ Cinnamon

☐ Fresh black pepper

☐ Garlic powder

☐ Basil

☐ Oregano

☐ Mustard

- ☐ BBQ sauce
- ☐ Ketchup
- ☐ Light mayonnaise
- ☐ Organic honey
- ☐ Truvia (or sweetener of choice)
- ☐ Aluminum foil
- ☐ Small, medium, and large size reusable plastic containers

---

- ☐ Eggs (organic)
- ☐ Milk (skim, soy, almond, or flaxseed)
- ☐ Mozzarella cheese
- ☐ Yogurt (3 nonfat 6 oz)

- ☐ Bran muffins (2)
- ☐ Whole wheat double fiber bread

- ☐ Apples (organic)
- ☐ Bananas
- ☐ Cantaloupe chunks
- ☐ Pineapple chunks
- ☐ Watermelon chunks

- ☐ Asparagus
- ☐ Baked potato/sweet potato (2)
- ☐ Celery sticks
- ☐ Cucumbers (1)

- ☐ Onion chopped (2 containers)
- ☐ Romaine lettuce (2 packages)
- ☐ Spinach
- ☐ Tomatoes (5)
- ☐ White mushrooms

- ☐ Albacore tuna (1 can)
- ☐ Chicken breast
- ☐ Roast beef (¼ lb sliced)
- ☐ Salmon
- ☐ Tilapia
- ☐ Turkey breast (¼ lb sliced)
- ☐ Turkey burgers (extra lean)

- ☐ Baked cheddar goldfish crackers
- ☐ Cashews raw no salt
- ☐ Kashi Bars (Chewy Granola)
- ☐ Kashi Chocolate Soft – Baked Squares
- ☐ Oatmeal cookies (Back to Nature)
- ☐ Pretzels 100 calorie pack
- ☐ Weight Watchers Ice Cream Bars

WEEK 8 DAY 1

BREAKFAST
1 bran muffin
6 cantaloupe chunks
1 cup milk
1 cup coffee or tea
1 cup water

SNACK
6 oz nonfat yogurt
1 cup water

LUNCH
Grilled chicken sandwich on whole wheat bun
Lettuce, tomato, and onion
Mustard, ketchup, or light mayonnaise
¼ bottle light cranberry juice and ¾ bottle water

SNACK
Pretzels 100 calorie pack
1 cup water

DINNER
4 oz baked chicken
½ baked or sweet potato
½ plate steamed spinach
1 bottle water

DESSERT
1 Weight Watchers ice cream bar
1 cup milk

WEEK 8 DAY 2

BREAKFAST
1 minute egg sandwich (recipe on page 97)
6 watermelon chunks
1 cup milk
1 cup coffee or tea
1 cup water

SNACK
1 Kashi Chewy Granola bar
1 cup water

LUNCH
2 slices roast beef on 1 slice whole wheat double fiber bread
Mustard, ketchup, or light mayonnaise
1 bottle water

SNACK
1 package baked cheddar goldfish crackers
1 cup water

DINNER
Turkey burger on whole wheat bun
Lettuce, tomato, and onion
Mustard, ketchup, or light mayonnaise
Medium-large salad with 1 tbsp light salad dressing
1 bottle water

DESSERT
1 Kashi Chocolate Soft Baked Square
1 cup milk

WEEK 8 DAY 3

BREAKFAST

Wheatena toasted wheat cereal (1 serving) add 1 tbsp ground flaxseeds and sweetener
6 pineapple chunks
1 cup milk
1 cup coffee or tea
1 cup water

SNACK

6 oz nonfat yogurt
1 cup water

LUNCH

Tuna and tomato wheel (recipe on page 98)
Tomato, onion, and cucumber salad (recipe on page 99)
1 bottle water

SNACK

2 oatmeal cookies
1 cup water

DINNER

Baked tilapia with seasoned bread crumbs
½ cup brown rice
½ plate steamed white mushrooms
¼ bottle light cranberry juice and ¾ bottle water

DESSERT

1 Weight Watchers ice cream bar
1 cup milk

WEEK 8 DAY 4

BREAKFAST

½ cup low-fat granola Heartland

6 cantaloupe chunks

1 cup coffee or tea

1 cup water

SNACK

10 raw cashews

1 cup water

LUNCH

½ peanut butter and honey sandwich

1 apple

1 bottle water

SNACK

Pretzels 100 calorie pack

1 cup water

1 cup green tea for energy boost

DINNER

Chicken Parmesan (recipe on page 101)

½ cup whole grain pasta with ½ cup tomato sauce

Medium-large salad with 1 tbsp extra virgin olive oil
and rice vinegar

1 bottle water

DESSERT

200 calorie milkshake (recipe on page 103)

WEEK 8 DAY 5

BREAKFAST
1 bran muffin
½ banana
1 cup milk
1 cup coffee or tea
1 cup water

SNACK
½ banana
5 raw cashews
1 cup water

LUNCH
½ turkey sandwich
1 apple
1 bottle water

SNACK
1 package of baked cheddar goldfish crackers
1 cup water

DINNER
4 oz broiled salmon
½ baked or sweet potato
½ plate steamed asparagus
1 bottle water

DESSERT
2 oatmeal cookies
1 cup milk

WEEK 8 DAY 6

BREAKFAST

    2 egg whites scrambled

    1 slice toast

    6 watermelon chunks

    1 cup coffee or tea

    1 cup water

SNACK

    1 Kashi chewy Granola bar

    1 cup water

LUNCH

    ½ roast beef sandwich

    Medium-large salad with 1 tbsp light salad dressing

    1 bottle water

SNACK

    10 raw cashews

    1 cup water

DINNER

    4 oz lean beef sirloin

    ½ baked or sweet potato

    ½ plate spinach, mushrooms, and onions (sauté in small amount of extra virgin olive oil)

    1 bottle water

DESERT

    1 Kashi Chocolate Soft Baked Square

    1 cup milk

WEEK 8 DAY 7

BREAKFAST

Cinnamon French Toast (recipe on page 98)
6 pineapple chunks
1 cup milk
1 cup coffee or tea
1 cup water

SNACK

10 cashews
1 cup water

LUNCH

Egg salad sandwich (recipe on page 101)
10 celery sticks with 1 tbsp light salad dressing
1 bottle water

SNACK

6 oz nonfat yogurt
1 cup water

DINNER

4 oz grilled tuna steak
½ cup brown rice
½ plate boiled green beans
1 bottle water

DESSERT

2 oatmeal cookies
1 cup milk

Now repeat the diet!

Work Out Program

Warm-up Exercises

1. Shoulder stretch

Sit on gluteus and put arms behind you. Move forward until you feel stretch in the shoulders. Hold position for 60 seconds. This exercise stretches the deltoid muscle. Photographs show front and lateral views.

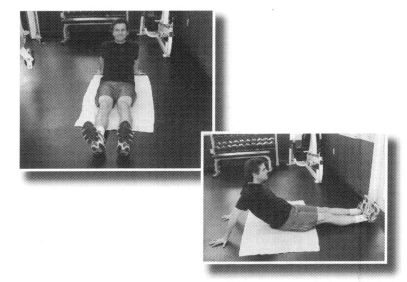

2. Lumbar and gluteus stretch

Lie on your back and bring left foot to right hand. Hold this position for sixty seconds. Switch sides with right foot to left hand. Again hold for sixty seconds. This will stretch both the lower back and the hips. Please see both photos.

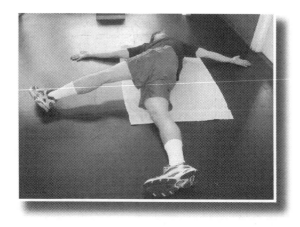

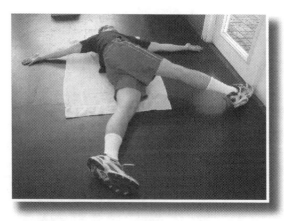

3. Hurdler stretch for hamstrings and quadriceps

Get into a position as if you were jumping a hurdle. Lean forward and try and touch your left foot with your left hand. Hold position for sixty seconds. Lie back and hold this position for sixty seconds

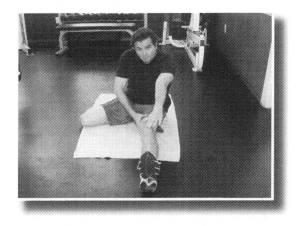

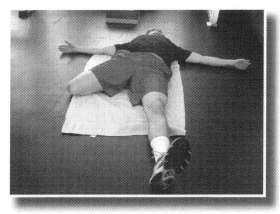

Switch to the other leg and repeat. Reach for the right foot with the right hand. Hold position for sixty seconds. Lie back and hold this position for sixty seconds. Total time for this stretch is four minutes.

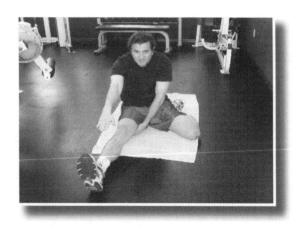

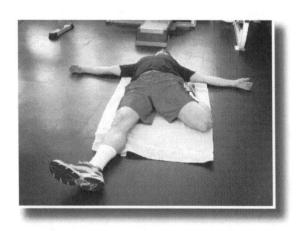

4. Lumbar stretch

Sit on floor and roll backward. Bring your legs over your head. Hold this position for sixty seconds. This will stretch your lower back. Be careful not to strain your neck.

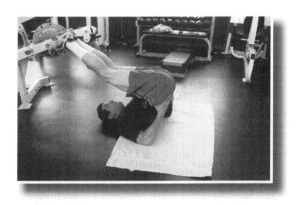

5. Butterfly stretch

Sit on the floor. Bring your feet toward your groin and gently press your knees downward. Press your elbows against your upper legs. Hold this position for 60 seconds. This exercise stretches your groin muscles.

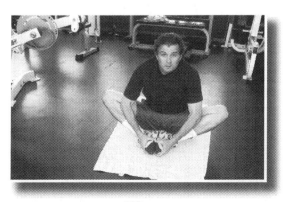

6. Crunches

Lie down on the floor. Bend your legs so your knees are up. Put your hands behind your head. Be careful not to pull on your neck. Lift your shoulder blades off the floor. This will tighten your abdominal muscles. This is good for your core. Do three sets of thirty.

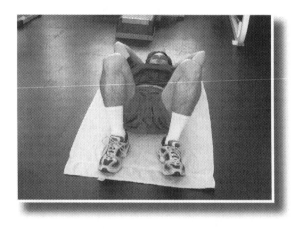

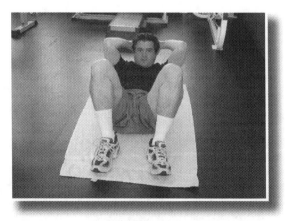

7. Push ups

Lie in prone position on the floor. Put your hands apart where you feel comfortable. Keep your feet together. Push your body up with your arms. This exercise warms up chest, shoulders, triceps, and biceps. Do three sets of fifteen reps.

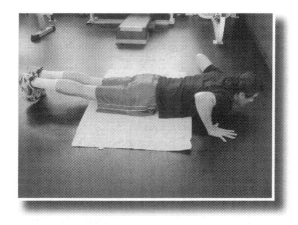

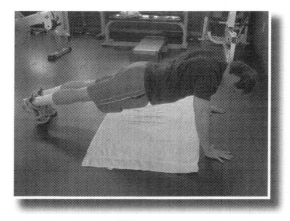

Cardiovascular Exercise

Chose one exercise and stay with it.

1. One hour of walking

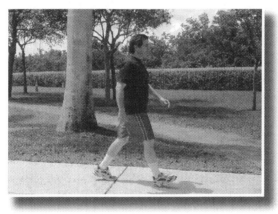

2. One hour of run-walk-run

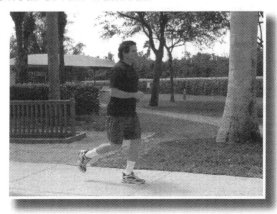

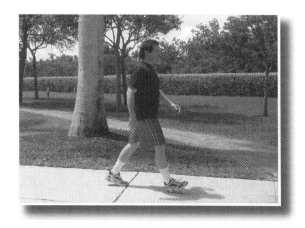

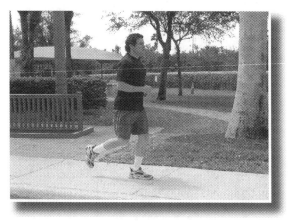

3. One hour of biking

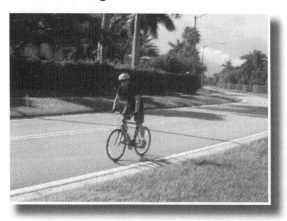

4. One hour of rollerblading

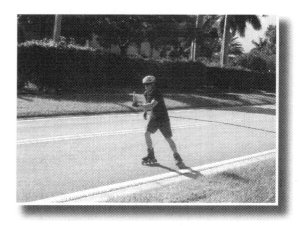

5. One hour of swimming

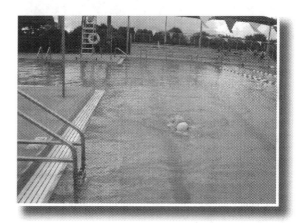

6. One hour of walking in a pool, aqua aerobics, or diving

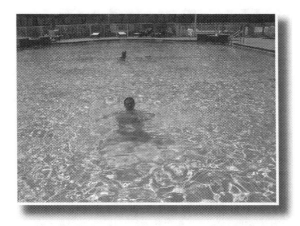

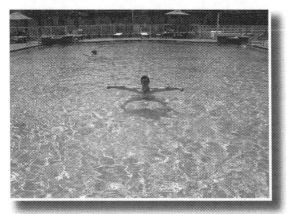

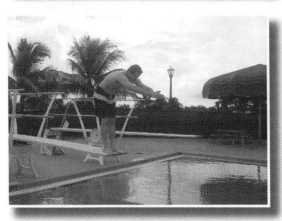

7. One hour of treadmill, elliptical, or stationary bike.

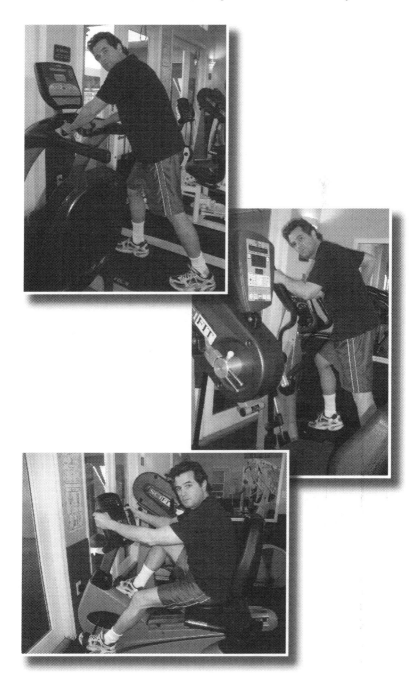

Cool Down

Do one to five minutes of the chosen exercise at a slower pace to cool down, or repeat the stretching exercises.

Note: Before starting any vigorous exercise program, please consult with your doctor. If you reach a plateau, do cardiovascular exercise for an hour and a half. Remember to gradually increase to this level.

Restaurants

America is a great, big melting pot. We are a nation of multiple ethnic groups from all over the world. When eating out, it is always fun to try different ethnic foods. These ethnic foods have now become part of the American diet. The following is a list of a few of my favorite restaurants located in South Florida, where I live, with examples of what you can order and how much. You can order similar dishes at your favorite local restaurants where you live. Bon Appetite!

Café Prima Pasta (Italian)

414 71st St
Miami Beach, FL 33141
(305) 867-0106
Order: Prima Salad with dressing on the side and Pollo Marsalla (eat ½ order).
Drink: 1 glass white wine and 1 glass water with lemon
Web: www.primapasta.com

Specchio Italian Café and Restaurant (Italian)

9485 Harding Ave
Surfside, FL 33154
(305) 865-5653
Order: Mixed salad with light dressing on the side and Gnocchi with Pomodoro sauce (eat ½ order).

Drink: 1 glass red wine and 1 glass water with lemon
Web: Google Specchio Italian Restaurant

Capital Grill – Miami (Steak House)

444 Brickell Avenue
Miami, FL 33131
(305) 374-4500
Order: Chopped salad with light dressing on the side. Kona Sirloin without bone or butter (eat ½ of steak only). For side dish, order baked potato (eat only ½) and grilled asparagus.
Drink: 1 glass red wine and 1 glass water with lemon
Web: www.capitalgrill.com

The Palms (Steak House)

9650 East Bay Harbor Drive
Bay Harbor Island, FL 33154
(305) 868-7256
Order: Mixed green salad with garlic vinaigrette on the side. Filet Mignon or prime New York Strip (eat ½). Baked potato (eat ½) and green beans.
Drink: 1 glass red wine and 1 glass water with lemon.
Web: www.thepalm.com

Joe's Stone Crab (Seafood)

11 Washington Ave
Miami Beach, FL 33139
(305) 673-0365
Order: Chopped salad with Joe's vinaigrette on the side. 1 order of Jumbo Stone crabs with side of mustard sauce. Add 1 pumpernickel and onion dinner role.
Drink: 1 ultra-light beer and 1 glass water with lemon.
Dessert: Key Lime pie (eat only ½) and 1 cup coffee.
Web: www.joesstonecrab.com

Captain Jim's Seafood

12950 W Dixie Highway

North Miami, FL 33161

(305) 867-0106

Order: 3 jumbo stone crabs with side of mustard sauce. Steamed vegetables and ½ order of mashed potatoes.

Drink: Ultra-light beer and 1 glass water with lemon

Web: Google Captain Jim's Seafood menu

Thai House II (Thai and Japanese)

2250 NE 163rd street

North Miami Beach, FL 33160

(305) 940-6075

Order: Thai salad with peanut dressing on the side. Seafood combination with brown rice (eat ½), or Miso soup with edamame. Sushi roll with brown rice.

Drink: Green tea

Web: www.thaihouse2.com

Epicure Gourmet Market and Café

17190 Collins avenue

Sunny Isles Beach, FL 33160

(305) 947-4581

Order: specialty soups from prepared food section and incorporate into diet plan.

Web: www.epicuremarket.com

Mo's Bagels and Deli (American Delicatessen)

2780 NE 187th St

Aventura, FL 33180

(305) 936-8555

Order: Vegetable soup, tuna fish on whole wheat bagel with lettuce, tomato, and onion (eat ½).
Drink: Bottle water or Dr. Brown's diet soda.

Shalom Haifa (Israeli)

18533 West Dixie Highway
North Miami Beach, FL 33183
(305) 936-1800
Order: Israeli salad, Chicken Shashlik with rice and beans (eat ½). Take out order of chicken soup.
Drink: 1 glass white wine and 1 glass water with lemon.
Dessert: Bavarian Cream pie (share with 2 or 3 people)
Web: www.Shalomhaifa.com/

Char-Hut (American Grill)

Multiple locations
9000 W SR 84
Davie, FL 33324
(954) 474-9312
Order: Large salad with light salad dressing on the side and Char-chicken or Char-tuna on whole wheat bun. Add all vegetables and hot sauce on the side.
Drink: Bottle water
Web: www.charhut.com

Padrino's Cuban Cuisine

Multiple locations
2500 E Hallandale Beach Blvd
Hallandale, FL 33009
(954) 456-4550
Order: Bistec de Pollo (grilled chicken with onions) with white rice, black beans, and sweet plantains (eat ½).

Drink: 1 glass sangria and 1 glass water with lemon.

Web: www.padrinos.com

Flanigan's (Seafood and American Fare)

Multiple locations
9516 Harding Ave (Surfside Plaza)
Surfside, FL 33154
(305) 867-0099
Order: Dinner salad with light dressing on the side. Fresh tuna with baked potato (eat ½).

Drink: Ice tea with lemon (no sugar) add sweetener.

Web: www.flanigans.com

Product List

1. Kashi Bar, Kashi Go Lean Crunch Cereal and Kashi Chocolate Square www.kashi.com
2. Quaker Oatmeal www.quakeroats.com
3. Truvia www.truvia.com
4. Smucker's Organic peanut butter www.smuckersnaturalpeanutbutter.com
5. Smart Balance Smart'n Healthy popcorn www.smartbalance.com
6. Chips Ahoy Reduced Fat cookies www.nabiscoworld.com/chipsahoy/
7. Jala Bars probiotic low fat frozen yogurt and fudge bars www.jalabars.com
8. Weight Watchers Diet Brownies and Chocolate Ice Cream Bars www.weightwatchers.com
9. Oreo Cookies Reduced fat www.nabiscoworld.com/brands/productinformation.aspx?...oreo...
10. Pringles potato chips 100 calorie pack www.fatsecret.com>foods>brandlist>pringles
11. Doritos 100 calorie pack www.fritolay.com/our.../doritos-nacho-cheesecal-minis.html
12. Vitamin water Zero www.glaceau.com
13. Eddy's frozen coconut fruit bars www.edy's.com
14. Centrum Vitamins www.centrum.com
15. Heartland low fat granola cereal www.heartlandgranola.com
16. Cream of Wheat Enriched Farina www.creamofwheat.com
17. Wheatena toasted wheat cereal www.wheatena.com
18. Back to Nature Oatmeal Cookies www.backtonature.com
19. 100 calorie pack pretzels www.snydersofhanover.com
20. Goldfish Crackers in Multi-packs (Baked Cheddar) www.pepperridgefarm.com
21. Pam Non-Stick Cooking Spray www.pamcookingspray.com
22. Smart Balance Non-Stick Cooking spray www.smartbalance.com

Bibliography

The Ten Golden Keys to Diet Success

1. Mosby's Medical Dictionary, 7th edition, St Louis: Elsevier, 2006
2. Webster's Ninth New Collegiate Dictionary, Springfield: Merriam – Webster Inc., 1983

Alarming Numbers

1. "American Heart disease Burden" Centers for Disease Control and Prevention, March 23, 2012, http://www.cdc.gov/heart disease/facts.htm/
2. "High Blood Pressure Frequently Asked Questions" Centers for Disease Control and Prevention, March 13, 2012, http://www.cdc.gov/blood pressure/faqs.htm
3. "Leading Causes of Death "Centers for Disease Control and Prevention, January 27, 2012, http://www.cdc.gov/nchs/fastats/lcod.htm/
4. "Top 10 Cancers Among Men" Centers for Disease Control and Prevention, June 22, 2011, http://www.cdc.gov/features/ds Men Top 10 Cancers
5. "Cancer Among Women" Centers for Disease Control and Prevention, May 1, 2012, http://www.cdc.gov/cancer/dcpc/data/women.htm
6. "Cancer and Men" Centers for Disease Control and Prevention, June 18, 2012, http://www.cdc.gov/features/cancerandmen/
7. "Adult Obesity Facts" Centers for Disease Control and Prevention, April 27, 2012, http://www.cdc.gov/obesity/data/adult.html/
8. "Childhood Overweight and Obesity" Centers for Disease Control and Prevention, April 27, 2012, http://www.cdc.gov/obesity/childhood/index.html
9. "Diabetes Research and Statistics" Centers for Disease Control and Prevention, February 16, 2012, http://www.cdc.gov/diabetes/consumer/research.htm
10. " The Numbers Count : Mental Disorders in America" The National Institute of Mental Health http://www.nimh.gov/health/publications/the-numbers-count-mental-disorders-in-america/index.shtml
11. "Osteoarthritis and you" Centers for Disease Control and Prevention, February 9, 2012, http://www.cdc.gov/features/osteo arthritisplan

12. http://arthritis.about.com/od/painmanage/ss/painqa-2.htm, Carol Eustice, Guide to Arthritis Pain, October 18, 2011

13. Jackman, Robert, Purvis, Janey, Mallet, Barbara, " Chronic Non-malignant Pain in Primary Care" American Family Physician, November 15, 2008 78 (10): 1155-1162

Eat Less and Age Slower

1. Sears, Barry, Lawrence, Bill. Enter The Zone. New York: Harper-Collins, 1995

2. Mosby's Medical Dictionary, 7th edition, St Louis: Elsevier, 2006

Hormones

1. Sears, Barry, Lawrence, Bill. Enter The Zone. New York: Harper-Collins, 1995

Exercise: Get Into a Routine and Stay with It

1. Atkins, Robert C. Dr. Atkins New Diet Revolution. New York: Avon Books, an Imprint of Harper Collins Publishers, 1992

Exercise and Feel Great

1. http://en.Wikipedia.org/wiki/Endorphin.From Wikipedia, the free encyclopedia (Endorphin). July 31, 2012

Exercise and the Scientific Data

1. Audio-Digest Family Practice: Geriatric Care: Enhancing the Quality of Life/ Healthy Aging and Life Transitions Volume 60, Issue 28. E Lee Rice, D.O., July 28, 2012.

The Boxers and the Referee

1. http://en.Wikipedia.org/wiki/weight_class_(boxing)weight class(boxing)-Wikipedia, the free encyclopedia, October 12, 2011.

The Basics

1. http://www.uptodate.com. Graham A Colditz, MD, Dr. PH, Health Diet in Adults Sept 16, 2011

2. http://www.nal.usda.gov/fnicFpyr/pmap1.gif

Filling Up With Fruits and Vegetables

1. http:// www. WebMD. Com/diet/Volumetrics-what-it-is Kathleen M. Zelman, MPH, RD, LD, January 30, 2012

2. Glassman, Keri. The O2 Diet. New York: Rodale Inc., 2010

Liquids

1. http://ga.water.usgs.gov/edu/propertyyou.htmlwaterproperties: The water in you (Water Science for Schools), April 18, 2012
2. Agatston, Arthur. The South Beach Diet. New York: Random House, 2003.

Your Plate

1. http://diet.lovetoknow.com/wiki/What_is_the_Philosophy_of_the_Jenny_Craig_Diet. Kathleen Roberts What Is the Philosophy of the Jenny Craig Weight Loss Program? July 16, 2012.

Body Mass Index

1. http://www.en.wikepedia.org/wiki/Body_mass_index.Bodymass index Wikipedia, the free encyclopedia, February 20, 2012.
2. Glassman, Keri. The 02 Diet. New York: Rodale Inc., 2010

Glycemic Index

1. http://en.wikipedia.org/wiki/glycemic_indexGlycemicindex-Wikipedia, the free encyclopedia, February 21, 2012

Vitamins and Medication

1. Roizen, Michael F and Oz, Mechmet C. You On a Diet. New York: Free Press A Division 0f Simon and Schuster, Inc., 2006 and 2009.
2. Monthly Prescribing Reference (MPR), December 2012, Volume 28, Number 12, Haymarket Media Inc., New York

Looking at Labels

1. Gonzalez, Tony and Dulan, Mitzi. The All-Pro Diet. New York: Rodale Inc., 2009